INTRODUCTION TO
YOGA
PRINCIPLES AND
PRACTICES

INTRODUCTION TO
YOGA
PRINCIPLES AND
PRACTICES

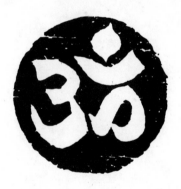

SACHINDRA KUMAR MAJUMDAR

THE CITADEL PRESS   SECAUCUS, N.J.

First paperbound printing, 1976
Copyright © 1964 by Sachindra Kumar Majumdar
All rights reserved
Published by Citadel Press
A division of Lyle Stuart, Inc.
120 Enterprise Ave., Secaucus, N.J. 07094
In Canada: George J. McLeod Limited, Toronto
Manufactured in the United States of America
ISBN 0-8065-0542-7

TO

The great sons of India who discovered at the
dawn of civilization the immortal Truth of Spirit
through their concrete life, critical thought, dominant self-will and heroic self-denial; who saw the
unity of existence behind the plurality of manifestation; and who formulated for the first time
in history the true principles of the Freedom and
Equality of Man.

CONTENTS

FOREWORD　　　　　　　　　　　　　　　　　11

I. PERSPECTIVE　　　　　　　　　　　　　　19

THE UPANISHADS　　　　　　　　　　　　　22
THE YOGA SUTRAS　　　　　　　　　　　　23
SOCIETY: THE HINDU AND THE GREEK　　　24
ORIGINS　　　　　　　　　　　　　　　　　30
YOGA AND LIFE AND WORLD　　　　　　　34
YOGA AND ASCETICISM　　　　　　　　　　36
YOGA AND PERSONALITY　　　　　　　　　39
YOGA AND SOCIETY　　　　　　　　　　　　40
YOGA AND BUDDHISM　　　　　　　　　　　43
YOGA AND HINDUISM　　　　　　　　　　　46
EAST AND WEST　　　　　　　　　　　　　　48

II. PRINCIPLES　　　　　　　　　　　　　　53

YOGA AND POWER　　　　　　　　　　　　　56
YOGA, EXISTENTIALISM AND ZEN　　　　　60
MIND AND FORMS OF AWARENESS　　　　　66
CONCENTRATION AND SAMADHI　　　　　　67
YOGA AS AWAKENING　　　　　　　　　　　68
LIFE AND EVOLUTION　　　　　　　　　　　69
PURPOSE IN LIFE　　　　　　　　　　　　　72
TRUTH AND ILLUSION　　　　　　　　　　　74
SPIRIT AND NATURE , GUNAS, EVOLUTION　78
MAN, HIS BONDAGE AND FREEDOM　　　　85
KARMA AND REBIRTH　　　　　　　　　　　88
ACTION AND FREEDOM　　　　　　　　　　95

III. PRACTICE: HATHA YOGA　　　　　　　99

HATHA YOGA IN MODERN INDIA AND THE WEST　　102
THE TECHNIQUES AND GENERAL FACTORS OF HEALTH　105
FOOD, FAST AND ASCETICISM　　　　　　　112
GENERAL REMARKS ABOUT YOGA EXERCISES　　129

BREATHING 130
POSTURES 139
MUDRAS AND BANDHAS OR SPECIAL TECHNIQUES 173
CLEANSINGS 174
ABDOMINO-RECTI MUSCLE CONTROL 178
TRATAKA AND KAPALABHATI 180
GLANDS AND YOUTHFULNESS 181
ORDER OF EXERCISES 182

IV. PRACTICE: MEDITATION 187

RAJA YOGA: CLASSIFICATION AND DEFINITION OF TERMS 187
PRACTICE 190
PRANAYAMA 198
THE KUNDALINI AND THE CHAKRAS 205
MEDITATION ON FINE SENSE PERCEPTION 210
MEDITATION ON DREAM EXPERIENCES 211
MEDITATION AND HEALTH 213
DRUG EXPERIENCE AND SAMADHI 217
ETHICS 221

V. SELECTIONS 231

THE VEDAS AND THE UPANISHADS 231
THE GITA 259

SELECT BIBLIOGRAPHY 295
GLOSSARY OF SANSKRIT WORDS 299
INDEX 307

ILLUSTRATIONS

BREATHING, ABDOMINAL-RIBCAGE 132
PERFECT POSTURE (SIDDHASANA) 140
LOTUS POSTURE (PADMASANA) 142
THE COBRA POSE (BHUJANGASANA) 143
THE LOCUST:POSE (SHALABHASANA) 144
THE BOW POSE (DHANURASANA) 145
BACK-STRETCHING POSE (PASCHIMOTTANA ASANA) 146
PANPHYSICAL POSE (SARVANGASANA) 147
PLOW POSE (HALASANA) 148
THE FISH POSTURE (MATSYASANA) 149
THE WHEEL (CHAKRASANA) 150
THE CAMEL POSE (USHTRASANA) 151
PELVIC POSE (SUPTA-VAJRASANA) 152
THE PEACOCK POSE (MAYURASANA) 153
HEAD STAND (SHIRSHASANA) 154
HEADKNEE BEND (PADAHASTASANA) 156
HIP STAND 157
SPINAL SIDE TWISTS (ARDHA MATSYENDRASANA) 158
THE GREAT POSE (MAHAMUDRA) 160
TRIANGLE POSE (TRIKONASANA) 161
MOUNTAIN POSE (PARVATASANA) 162
YOGA MUDRA 163
KING OF DANCER'S POSE (NATARAJASANA) 164
ONE LEG STAND (EKAPADASANA) 165
HEADKNEE BEND (PADAHASTASANA) 165
BOUND LOTUS POSE (BADDHA PADMASANA) 166
HEADSTAND IN BOUND LOTUS (BADDHA PADMASANA SHIRSHASANA) 167
COCK POSE (KUKKUTASANA) 168
LATERAL SPINE POSTURE 1 (UTTITHA MERUDANDASANA) 169
LATERAL SPINE POSTURE 2 (UTTITHA MERUDANDASANA) 169
TREE POSE (VRIKSHASANA) 170
FORWARD HEAD-BEND (BHUNAMANASANA) 171
THE DEAD POSE (SHAVASANA)) 172
UDDIYANA) 178
NAULI 179
THE CHAKRAS 204

FOREWORD

Reason is inconclusive; the scriptures vary; there is no philosopher who does not differ from another. The truth of religion and ethics is hidden away in the hearts of men. That by which the great ones have traversed is the road.

THE MAHABHARATA (Hindu Epic, c.1500 B.C.)

IN THE FOLLOWING PAGES, I have tried to give the substance of yoga, its principles and practices, as they have come down to us from an immemorial past. As a teacher, I have long felt the need for a book which would present succinctly, to the general public, a subject which is daily becoming a matter of increasing interest in the West, but about which prejudice and misinformation abound.

It is my wish to present yoga as a living tradition, not as a system of fixed formulas, to be found in books or schools. Yoga is not a special religion or a particular philosophical doctrine. It is the wisdom of life. It is experience. Yoga and life do not stand apart or opposed to one another. Yoga is the intelligent and self-conscious effort of man towards achieving universal existence; that harmony between individual and cosmos which nature, herself, is subconsciously striving toward through trial, error and waste.

We search for truth on two levels; one physical, the other spiritual. Science and wisdom are the fruits of this search. We seek to know the underlying facts and principles of nature. We desire to understand the goals of our own lives. In truth, we have need of both science and wisdom to live a life that is rich and meaningful.

In this twofold search for truth, we start from our commonsense

11

perceptions and feelings. But as we proceed, our investigations throw doubt upon them. Science reveals that the notions which formed the starting point of our enquiry are superficial and illusory in character due to the natural limitation of our senses. In the same manner, wisdom and maturity reveal that our everday ideas and feelings about the self, the personality and its goals, are not the deepest or most constant truths of our nature. The obvious is not the profound. This judgement about the ephemeral and superficial character of our ordinary feelings and perceptions stems from a deeper and more enduring experience which contradicts them. The experience of wisdom is final. When the light of Truth shines, all illusions vanish for good.

The highest truth of self or spirit is an experience and an indubitable fact, yet when we try to express it in words, we are handicapped by the natural inadequacy of language.

Language is symbolic. Words are names for experience. They are a means to communication and action; useful and practical. But words are not facts. Statements are imperfect representations of truth. A statement, even in its symbolic sense, is significant, true or false, only in a context which is dynamic in the world. No sooner do we make a statement then we notice the qualifications it needs. The only sure, clear and absolutely valid statements are mathematical formulas and equations. But these are formal and tautological, empty and timeless, above all actual processes. In the concrete and dynamic situations of life, statements can only have relative significance.

When we come to the highest yogic experience of Pure Consciousness and Selfhood beyond all duality, language loses all power of expression. Therefore, it has been said in the Kena Upanishad, (c. 1000 B.C.); the Self is one "from which words recoil along with the mind without ever grasping it." Silence is more eloquent of wisdom than words. This is the yoga view of truth, language and experience. Yet yoga must make use of language and logic to help men see that the integral experience of Truth that lies beyond reason is not its denial but the fulfilment of its ideals. Words must point the way.

People who have freed themselves from childish dreams and illusions, who have seen through the game of life, its joys and sorrows, successes and failures, loves and hates, follies and cruelties, have come to realize that life is lived mostly in ignorance. Man is out of touch with reality. He lives in false hopes and unjustifiable dreams and is bound, above all, in slavery to one thing or another. There can be no solution to the tragedy and enigma of existence, no realization of our idealistic aspirations, no redemption from evil, unless we find a higher truth. Yoga is the search for and the realization of this truth.

The highest truth of life is a spiritual experience; not an intellectual conception. This experience is wisdom, which is acquired through faith in human destiny and effort toward self-realization. Higher life is a matter of growth. Experience and thought are necessary to comprehend its meaning.

The search for wisdom or yoga will never be a mass movement. Neither are love and justice practiced en masse. Most people are too indolent to think or to act for themselves; they are governed and led predominantly by unenlightened drives. But those few who strive for higher truth are the lights who will guide their fellow men. They will inspire others with faith in the reality of those ideals which alone save life from pedestrian intellectualism, sightless rationalism, doubt, despair and ultimate tragedy.

In the Shvetashvatara Upanishad (c. 1000 B.C.), an ancient yoga text, it is said: "He who has supreme devotion to the Divine and the same to the teacher as to the Divine, to that great heart the truths spoken here will become manifest." The sense of this verse is that one who is dedicated to the ideals of truth, freedom and love, who is not misguided and corrupted by materialism, and is not disheartened by pain, disappointment, denial and doubt, will one day discover the great truths of the spirit in his own heart. Those who lift up their eyes — they alone see the heavens and the stars.

The trouble with many today is not that they have forgotten what happened in their early childhood and not that they lack instinctual satisfaction. They have lost their faith in the spiritual truth of man and, in so doing, have sacrificed their most valuable possession — their own creative power.

Yoga is practical psychology. It is a method of training the mind and developing its powers of subtle perception so that man may discover for himself the spiritual truths on which religious beliefs and moral values finally rest. Yoga is the realization of our hidden powers.

There is a widespread feeling today that science and scientific methods have severe limitations. They can tell us much about the world but are incapable of solving the specifically human problems of establishing values and forming character. We have need of another approach, another method to understand and resolve human conflicts and to master life. Our method must be both intelligent and rational, for it will be of no avail if we simply turn back to outworn creeds and superstitions.

Ever since biblical belief first confronted Greek reason, thinkers in the West have been perplexed by their inherent contradictions. Schools and systems of philosophy are replete with the various attempts to resolve those difficulties. Despite centuries of effort in that direction, however, no satisfying and enduring solution to the problem of reason and faith has emerged.

The spreading interest in yoga in the West today is due to the growing realization that it throws an entirely new light on the problems of practical psychology and spiritual philosophy, at the same time providing a unique method of self-development dedicated to self-realization. I hope the present book will meet this need and introduce the student to the essential truths of yoga. Thereafter, he can proceed to further study and investigation equipped with a clearer understanding of yoga's basic ideas and aims.

To this end, I have divided the book into four sections. In the first, I have provided a perspective for the better understanding of yoga through an examination of its history and development, as well as through discussion of yoga's relationship to many different aspects of life. The second section deals with basic ideas and principles of yoga. The third section is devoted to methods of yoga practice and the subject of meditation. This division gives an overall account of hatha yoga and an intimate glimpse into the lives and practices of ascetics in the deep interior of the Himalayas. The last section of the book contains a rich selection of yoga literature dating from the earliest to most recent times. I have included a glossary of Sanskrit words which I hope will be helpful to the reader.

I
PERSPECTIVE

I
PERSPECTIVE

AN INTRODUCTION TO YOGA

YOGA IS ESSENTIALLY practice and experience. It is the practice of inwardness and silent meditation; it is the experience of perfect calmness of mind and self-knowledge. Yoga is an art, a technique for achieving the purest form of Self-awareness devoid of all thought and sensation. Such knowledge of Self has the power to destroy illusions about our nature and the world, and thus release us from the bondage of fear and ignorance. Truth makes us free — the fundamental truth of existence. Yoga is the highest wisdom; it is the most perfect form of Self-expression.

Yoga is the art of life. Art achieves practical results through both theory and practice; art as technique needs conceptions and ideas to guide it in the achievement of its goal. Yoga, as the art of living, has its formulations, its interpretations of life, based upon subtle perceptions gained through concentration. These interpretations are not the supreme silent truth that is beyond speech and mind, but they do give us a picture of the subtle realities of life and help us to live intelligently. They are conceptions which illuminate our life and moral sense, our activity and spiritual aspiration, our quest for truth, goodness, beauty and perfection. They provide the deepest insight into the profound mystery of existence and guide life to its fulfillment.

Our knowledge of the world is a series of groping interpretations. It will never be complete. The mind will be forever formulating its experiences in new ways. But the mind has boundaries which reason and sense cannot overleap. Existence or truth as *fact* is known directly through yogic superconsciousness, which alone can penetrate the mind's barriers. In that realm, the limitations of sense and logical reasoning are left behind and consciousness reveals itself in its pristine purity. The ultimate questions of life, the undying queries of man are answered and the most profound stirrings of the heart realized in the supreme silence of wisdom. For the one who has had this experience, there is no need to seek elsewhere. For others, still bound by sense and reason, the mystery and search remain forever tantalizing and unfulfilled. But truth is waiting in every heart and will be revealed to him who has tired of the search without and chooses to look within.

Yoga as a living tradition of thought, practice and culture has never been contained in any book. It is not a closed system. Systems are great achievements of mind, attempts of reason to give a clear, consistent and complete picture of existence. But those who know enough do not make systems. Systems throw light here and there and make more or less sense insofar as they reflect the realities of life as seen through a consistent point of view. But doubts remain, falsities linger and dark corners abound. If, however, a thought structure touches our mind and heart deeply, because we recognize therein a relation to the truths of life, it will retain its hold on us and continue to govern us in our conduct. Yoga is more than an intellectual conception of truth; it is perception (*darshana*) itself. The yoga books themselves tell us to go beyond books and formulas, personalities and beliefs, to recognize no other authority than one's inmost self, the supreme teacher of all, and to accept no rule or command which goes against the truth of one's own nature. Yoga is the religion of man.

It will be helpful here if we briefly explore the background of yoga and the context in which it arose in ancient India. This will provide a useful perspective, help relate yoga to the life of today and allow us to consider several questions which arise to trouble the modern mind.

The yogic tradition began in northern India at least five thousand years ago among a people who called themselves *Aryans* (noblemen) and *Dvijas* (twice-born). The Dvijas considered themselves to be twice-born: first, naturally, and second, spiritually, when at an early age, they were initiated into the life of worship, prayer and meditation. Dvija originally meant "bird". The bird is considered to be twice-born: first in the shell, and second into the freedom of the sky when the shell is broken. So also might a man be born into the freedom of the spirit when all wordly illusions had fallen away.

Later, yoga spread to other Indian peoples who came to be assimilated into a single society despite the differences of race and culture.

Yoga is clearly mentioned in the oldest literature of the Aryan, or Indo-European people. This literature, called the *Vedas* (knowledge), is comprised of both poetry and prose. It is very extensive and represents the growth and development of a tradition over a period of thousands of years (from C.3,000 to 800 B.C., speaking conservatively). Much has been lost along the way, and the portions which have come down to us have been edited and compiled in their present form.

The vedic literature, composed in archaic Sanskrit, later came to be divided into four categories: *Samhitas* (hymns), *Brahmanas* (rituals and liturgy), *Aranyakas* (forest meditations), and the *Upanishads* (mystical and philosophical compositions). The Vedas as a whole are also divided into four groups: The *Rig Veda*, the *Sama Veda*, the *Yajur Veda* and the *Atharva Veda*. Each of the groups contains the four classes of literature mentioned above.

THE UPANISHADS

The *Upanishad* literally means the secret knowledge that is communicated from teacher to disciple — to the disciple who is fit to receive it. The Upanishads, which were the last books of the vedic literature to be composed and which represent the peak of vedic development, are the original source books of yoga. In the later post-vedic periods, many books came to be composed under the name of "Upanishads". But they do not enjoy the prestige and authority of the vedic Upanishads which are 10 to 13 in number. These were all composed before the time of the Buddha and are conservatively assigned to the period between 1200 and 800 B.C.

The Upanishads are also referred to as the Vedanta, i.e. the last part of the Vedas. Subsequently, Vedanta came to mean the philosophy, or the view of reality, to be found in the Upanishads. In later times, people differed in their interpretation and understanding of such views. Therefore, Vedanta came also to mean different schools of thought, intepretations, and ways of life based on the Upanishads. The Upanishads are mostly prophetic in character. They declare truth as experienced by men of supersensuous perception. They also give rational interpretations of their views, thus representing man's earliest attempt to understand and explain the world and life through reason and experience. The methods of directly perceiving truth are herein revealed. This is called *Adhyatma Yoga,* or that yoga which is the harnessing of the mind's powers so that man may concentrate those powers on his inmost self.

Yoga and Vedanta are not distinct outlooks and methods in the spiritual practice of India; they are one in actual life. Yoga is generally spoken of in the sense of practice, while Vedanta is specifically used to mean a conception of reality. Vedanta and yoga go together. Vedanta as merely an intellectual conception is lame. Yoga as pure activity is sightless. Practice is the essence of spiritual life, but it must always have a conception of the goal to lead it forward.

The Upanishads form a spiritual mine of inexhaustible significance. They have provided inspiration in every age and continue to shape Indian life and mind today. Their influence has quietly reached far beyond India's borders to distant lands. In the future, they will come to be the basis of faith for a vast portion of mankind.

While the Upanishads are the original source books of yoga, yoga teachings are to be found in many sections of the great Hindu epic, THE MAHABHARATA. The Gita, which forms a small part of this work, is a poetical composition of seven hundred verses which was written in pre-Buddhistic times, (before the 5th century B.C.). The Gita is the most popular Hindu scripture and gives the most universal expression to the spirit and fundamental concepts of yoga as *Brahma-vidya*, or the science of Brahman, i.e., Vedanta. Yoga teachings were later presented in organized form by many different schools, but most of their books have been lost. We often hear names of teachers whose compositions are no longer in existence, but fragments of whose writings remain, preserved in quotations by later authors and commentators.

THE YOGA SUTRAS

One of the comparatively late books, which has, for good reason, long been regarded as the outstanding compendium of yoga principles and practice, of yoga psychology, ethics, metaphysics and practice of concentration, is known as the YOGA SUTRAS OF PATANJALI or THE APHORISMS ON YOGA by Patanjali. This work is generally attributed to the third or second century B.C. Several commentaries on this book exist, among which Vyasa's is the oldest and most authoritative. Vyasa's work is the most profound philosophical work ever to have been written in Sanskrit, and is outstanding by reason of its scholarship, style, arrangement and depth. It belongs to the early centuries of the Christian era — not later than the fourth century A.D.

Both Patanjali's work and Vyasa's commentary have been translated into English. Patanjali's sutras have had many renderings. None of them are, however, completely satisfactory. Many key concepts and formulations remain unintelligible in these translations. Often the notes only serve to create further confusion. As time passed, philosophical learning, rationality and openness of mind declined in India for a variety of reasons. Many concepts became obscure and were overlaid with a veneer of superstition and dogma. Uncritical minds have made a caricature of yoga ideas and practices, producing many misunderstandings. Still there were always those who found their way to truth. Those few maintained the purity of yoga practice and view, and kept a sure hold on the essentials.

Today some kind of reconstruction of thought is necessary to understand clearly what the great yoga teachers of the past have taught. This requires practice and reflection, as well as study of the many concepts of yoga scattered in the philosophical literature of India, and familiarity with the spiritual discoveries of our own time.

Because of the prestige enjoyed by Patanjali's book and its wide circulation, there is a general misconception that yoga is based on his book. This is not so. Patanjali was not the founder of yoga. He was a most important systematizer. Belonging to one important school of yoga, he represents a view which is dualistic, and an attitude which is ascetic. A broader and more positive expression of yoga is found in the Upanishads, in the Gita and in a few other schools. The best minds of India have adhered to a broad, monistic and positive view, though they have given Patanjali due recognition for his marvelous systematization of yoga principles and practices.

SOCIETY: THE HINDU AND THE GREEK

Let us now turn our attention for a while to that civilization which gave rise to yoga. The ancient Indians, like the Greeks, were pioneers in civilization. Both were descended from a common stock. Their social and political institutions, their civilizations as pictured in the Homeric poems and the vedic literature, in the accounts of the Greek writers and historians of the pre-Christian centuries, all unmistakably point to this conclusion. The Aryans of India developed all the branches of study which the Greek cultivated — epic poetry, drama, philosophical literature, ethics, logic, metaphysics, mathematics, algebra, geometry, medicine, surgery, astronomy, astrology, music, sculpture and painting.

The Greeks were closer to the Orient than the Occident. The Greek people and civilization came from the East, from Asia Minor to Greece. The Greeks derived much of their art, science, religion and civilization from Egypt. The Egyptians who produced the great civilization of the Nile Valley came down from Punt, the upper reaches of the Nile. Historians of the Near and the Middle East, like H. R. Hall, have thought that the Egyptians came originally from India. The ancient Greeks were of the same origin as the ancient Persians and the Indo-Aryans. Ancient Greek, Latin, and Sanskrit are substantially the same language. The writings of Greek historians and biographers abound in acounts which connect India with Greece and which suggest that philosophers like Pythagoras, Democritus, Socrates and Plato were influenced by Indian and oriental thought.

The ideas and practices of sects like the Orphics and the Pythagoreans, and the opinions of philosophers like Empedocles, Heraclitus and Democritus remind us of India. The essence of Socratic and Platonic philosophy has remained unintelligible in the West because of lack of insight into Indian thought.

The Orphics believed, contrary to the popular Greek religion, in the divine essence of man, which is the teaching of the Upanishads. They and the Pythagoreans shared beliefs and practices which existed among several sects in vedic India. Plato's view of Reality is the same as that of the Upanishads. His method of attaining knowledge of the good is that of yoga. In the Phaedo, Plato describes silent meditation or inwardness as withdrawal of the senses from their objects and as stilling of the processes of mind. Only in this way, he says, can we know existence or truth as it is.

The Greek theoria of the Pythagoreans, of Socrates and Plato, from which the word "theater" comes, is the vision or *darshana* of the

Upanishads. Philosophic wisdom is *yogic prajna* (supersensuous knowledge) and not a speculative conclusion of reasoning.

Plato mentions in one of his letters that he has not written down the essence of his philosophy since true philosophic wisdom can only be communicated directly from teacher to disciple, like lighting one lamp by another. The Timaeus indicates that the receiver of truth must be a fit person — fit by character and not by reason of intellect alone. Reading Plato, one is constantly reminded of the Upanishads. Platonic thought is so un-Greek in the sense in which Greek thought is generally taken, namely, pure rationalism, that some philosophers, like Nietzsche, have called it "un-Hellenic."

Even Aristotle, the great rationalist and empiricist, upheld so strongly by teachers of philosophy in the West, is not fully understood. Aristotle speaks of intellect in the same sense as do the Upanishads — intellect which is not thinking logically, but which grasps truths immediately. Intellect, acording to him, knows through an intuitive, suprarational perception.

Aristotle talks of God-like contemplation as the highest and happiest activity of man. This is not thinking or reasoning but the direct, immediate apprehension of existence. His God is a self-contemplating Intelligence. Many teachers in the West, limited by a narrow naturalism and haunted by the dogmatic tradition of western religions, brush all this aside as a lingering Platonic fancy in Aristotle's mind. All this reminds one of the modern philosopher who remarked that philosophy is the finding of bad reasons for what one believes on instinct.

The thought of Plotinus is Hindu and has been recognized as such by many scholars in the West. Plotinus went with the Roman emperor Gordian to Persia in search of Indian wisdom. He studied long years in Egypt where teachers from India had given instruction centuries before his time.

The Greek and the Hindu were not only one people originally, but were in touch with one another long after their separation. The Persian empire brought the Greeks and the Indians close together.

Indian soldiers fought on Greek soil in the armies of the Persian emperors, Darius and Xerxes. Eusebius, in his biography of Socrates, relates an incident recorded in the fourth century B.C. in which Socrates met a brahmin in the *agora*, or market place. The brahmin asked Socrates what he was doing. Socrates replied that he was questioning people in order to understand man. At this the brahmin laughed and asked how one could understand man without knowing God.

The Socratic conceptions of freedom and virtue are those of the Upanishads. Socrates talked of the freeman, the autarch — the man who is not merely politically free, but who is self-ruled and self-governed. The Upanishadic word for autarch is *swatantra*, self-governed. The freeman is the ruler of himself — ruler of his body, senses and mind.

Socrates defined virtue as knowledge. Virtue is character, the realization of the essence of man. It is the knowledge of the Self of man; it is wisdom of the heart and not intellectual learning. This knowledge is the realization of the Apollonian dictum, *Know Thyself*, which is also the Upanishadic dictum, *Atmanam Viddhi*. In the Gita, knowledge or wisdom is defined as character. It is virtue i.e. manliness — manifestation of the essence of man. Virtue comes from the vedic word *vira* (hero), or man. A vedic prayer is for the manifestation of manliness — the universal man, the divine in man. This is the true basis of humanism.

Intellectuals have long pondered over the Socratic definition of virtue as knowledge, without being able to figure out precisely what it means.

The Orphic tradition of the divinity of man and the Socratic and Platonic view of life and reality did not strike deep roots in Greece. In India, the upanishadic culture continued to live despite the political and social vicissitudes of centuries. It has molded the life of India and has provided the basis for integrating an extraordinarily complex and pluralistic civilization of many races, languages and cultures. In recent times, the best minds of India — political, social, religious and cultural leaders — have all drawn inspiration from the Upanishads in their effort to integrate the priceless spiritual heritage of India with the scientific achievements of the West.

People often draw a radical distinction between cultures, between East and West and make sweeping generalizations. Truth is not so simple. When the Greeks first made the distinction between East and West, they meant by East, the Persians and by West, the Greeks — not the Europeans. Today, East and West have different meanings.

It is maintained that the West is scientific and the East is aesthetic; that there is some kind of radical difference between the West and the East in mind and character. There are obvious distinctions between races and nations, between cultures and civilizations. These distinctions have their use and importance. But the differences are not fundamental. We are all products of one life. In the universal march of life toward light and freedom, peoples and races, cultures and civlizations make their contributions at different periods of history. The same life, the same drive and urge, manifests and realizes itself differently in different circumstances.

No single people or nation has produced today's civilization. Peoples create, learn, borrow and recreate. When the creative urge is exhausted a civilization dies. The essence of a civilization lies in its spiritual outlook, its conception of human nature and freedom, human destiny and relationships. The material and scientific achievements of civilizations like the Greek and the Roman remain, as do the descendants of those people who once produced them. Yet we say that the civilizations are dead because their basic outlook on life, the spiritual view, is no longer the governing force of our time, but has been supplanted by a new conception. All talks of human excellence notwithstanding, the Greek civilization with its pride vanished for failure of insight into the essential truth of man.

Empires and kingdoms with all their might, pomp and pagaentry perish for lack of true vision. But the flowers of Spirit are deathless. "God grows weary of great kingdoms, but never of little flowers." (Tagore)

India was not less scientific or civilized than Greece. But her contribution to human civilization is still little known. Her thought has continued to influence the world from the most ancient times. The books of the Bible are not as original as they were once thought to be. The story of creation, of the flood, the Book of Deuteronomy, the Book of the Psalms, the parable of wisdom to be found in the Book of Solomon, have all been traced to Sumerian, Egyptian and Indian sources. The Essenes, forerunners of Christianity, bore clear influences of Indian spiritual thought and culture. There were Indian teachers in Asia Minor, in Greece, in Egypt — long before Christ. Many of the ideas and practices to be found in the Bible and in the Christian churches of later times derive from Indian sources. Logos, Father in Heaven (dyus pitar), non-resistance, renunciation and monasticism are all Indian ideas and practices.

Fifteen hundred years ago there was not much that might be called civilization in the forests of Western Europe. In the Middle Ages, the Arabs kept alive the learning of Greece and India. They communicated India's empirical medical tradition and decimal system of computation to Europe and the Italian universities and thus helped the growth of science in modern times.

Plato says in his dialogue Epinomis that whatever the Greeks have borrowed from non-Greeks they have carried to a higher perfection. So also the people of western Europe have carried to a superior excellence the things they have learned from earlier civilizations. Today, science and the free institutions of the West are travelling eastward. In the not too distant future, we may be surprised to witness new creative advances in knowledge and activity among peoples and nations who were once regarded as incapable of progress. There are ups and downs in the lives of nations as in the lives of individuals. The triumph of the moment counts little in the long run of things. In times to come, the world will be the home of a common humanity and civilization where distinctions based on ignorance and prejudice will disappear.

ORIGINS

Yoga arose in the age of the Vedas and Upanishads. It had its beginnings among a healthy, powerful and independent community which had attained a high level of culture. The founders of the tradition were drawn from learned and aristocratic families, from the scholars and warriors. The great prophets of India were kings and princes, leaders of thought and rulers of men. They had the best their time could offer in education and culture, in power and pleasure. But these thinkers and leaders came to grips with the fundamental questions and the ultimate concerns of men — the questions and concerns which press themselves on the attention of reflective and mature individuals. They examined life and sought its meaning and true goal. They saw the limitations of existence, its tragic reality, its dualities, the inevitable pain and suffering and the myraid illusions which surround life. They saw that our experiences in the world have meaning within limits, but do not invest life with the kind of significance the heart longs for. The realized that without such ultimate redeeming significance, the fragments of joy and sorrow, which weave like light and shadow through our life, are, in the long run absurd and pointless. This is the central problem of existence and the starting point of the existential search for the deeper truth which pure reason fails to discover. What is it that inspires man to heroic effort, to tireless striving for goodness, beauty, truth and justice, if the world is ruled by blind mechanical necessity and there is no concern in the heart of the universe for man, his values and aspirations?

These men realized their deep bond to humanity. They were moved by the suffering they saw around them and wanted to help man find freedom. They had attained the highest development of individuality through the discipline of reason and emotion, through the development of character. But they saw that although unique individuality is precious, its significance is limited by its obvious isolation and self-centeredness, and it can never encompass the total meaning of life.

True philosophy is a pragmatic search through understanding and effort for right values. It arises from the inescapable discontents and problems of life. Much in the same manner as did Freud in his book THE DISCONTENTS OF CIVILIZATION, the yoga teachers proclaimed that philosophical inquiry begins under the impact of threefold suffering in the realms of the natural, the social and the psychological. This discontent is existential.

That there is an answer to our search for truth and freedom and that there is a way to redeem our life from tragedy and pointlessness is a hope based on faith. But this hope and faith can only be verified by experience.

Faith in human freedom, perfectibility and redemption is natural to us, and is analogous to the faith on which science rests. Faith in the possibility of a rational order in the universe is the basis of science. It is a belief which has been increasingly verified by practice. Yet in the beginning there was nothing except hope to assure man that there was indeed such an order. The mind works that way. Verification comes later through observation and research.

In the same manner, the teachers of the Upanishads were inspired by the native hope and intuition of the human mind and sought the truth of life through reflection and inwardness. Truth comes through inquiry, practice and revelation.

In beautiful story and verse, the Upanishads relate to us how the search for spiritual truths began. We read in the Chhandogya Upanishad, for example, that Narada a man of vast scholarship approached a young saint, Sanat Kumara, and said that he knew all the branches of learning: the four Vedas, the ancient lore, grammar, mathematics, science of portents, science of time, logic, ethics and politics, theology, astronomy, fine arts and others. Yet he was no more than a knower of words because he did not know the Self. Narada had heard that those who know the Self cross over sorrow. Despite all his learning, he felt the tragedy of life and was seeking to overcome his sorrow. The young teacher imparted to him the higher knowledge of Reality.

In the Upanishads a distinction is made between two kinds of knowledge, the lower and the higher. Both are to be known. The lower knowledge concerns nature, phenomena, the many and the variable. The higher knowledge is about Brahman, the One, the Real and the Immutable.

Here we have a significant distinction between the knowledge of subject and the knowledge of object. Knowledge of object or nature is the knowledge of means. This helps us to attain our practical ends by giving us control over nature. It is useful, but does not help us distinguish right values or show us the true goal of life. Science gives us comfort, creates leisure and makes higher life possible, but it does not give us peace, happiness or true manhood. Knowledge of life's goal is to be sought deep within one's self through clarity of mind and calmness of heart.

A memorable verse in the Katha Upanishad proclaims: "The Self-Existent One *(causa sui)* made the senses outgoing; therefore they perceive external objects and not the Self within. But some rare sage, desirous of immortality, saw the inner Self with introverted vision." The teachers declare that they have known the Great Person, luminous like the sun, beyond darkness, and through Him have conquered death. They say that this person, the Divine Self, dwells always in the hearts of men, framed by thought, intelligence and mind. There is no other way to overcome the fear of death. They address men as heirs to immortal life.

This Self which remains hidden in the hearts of men cannot be known by one who is dull or restless, who is not strong, disciplined or self-controlled; it cannot be known by much learning or by reasoning. It can be known only through calmness of mind, through yoga, through contemplation. The Upanishads lay down three basic steps to this Self-realization. They are *shravana,* hearing, reading or instruction; *manana,* reflection or reasoning; and *nididhyasana;* meditation or contemplation.

The Self should be heard first. Then one should reflect upon what one has heard and try to understand what has been imparted. Finally, one should perceive the Self in silent meditation. Spiritual life is not intellectual death. Reasoning is an essential part of spiritual search, but spiritual perception is more than an abstract concept of the intellect.

Our spiritual ideal must make sense; it cannot be opposed to reason. The Hindu says, our God must grow. The God of a child is not the God of an adult; the God of the thinker or theologian is not the God of a man of spiritual perception. Our understanding of God improves with our growth; faith gets clarified and finally matures into experience. A popular Sanskrit verse declares: "Fire is the God of those who perform sacrifices; for the thinker God is in the heart; for men of small understanding God is in symbols; but for the Knowers the Divine is everywhere."

When people fight God, they fight their imaginations. They say God is dead; nothing is dead except their own childish notions.

The search for Self is a natural quest of man; it is the mainspring of human psychology — man's desire to know his true self and to discover his true identity. This is the natural religion, or the religion of man. There is in man an obvious and spontaneous desire for the pleasant as well. For the first time in the history of human thought, centuries before Plato, we find in the Upanishads a clear distinction drawn between the two ethical ideals, the pleasant and the good. Plato also talked of the natural appetite for pleasure and the acquired taste for the good. Many centuries later Kant was to make this concept the basis of his ethical discussion.

The Katha Upanishad declares that the man of wisdom examines both the pleasant and the good and makes the latter the supreme end. The man without discrimination chooses pleasure as the goal and perishes in his effort to attain it. A man who makes pleasure his ultimate goal is like an overgrown child for whom toys remain the all important things throughout life.

Man will never be satisfied with the passing, finite things of the world. His hunger is for the infinite (bhuma). The infinite is the true (Sat); it is the good (Shiva), it is also the purest delight (rasa), the essence of beauty.

YOGA AND LIFE AND WORLD

This is an appropriate moment to consider the attitude of yoga toward the world and worldly values. Many misconceptions prevail on the subject. Yoga is the art of living. Our life is given to us to live and not to suppress. It is up to us to live it sensibly and not to dissipate our forces stupidly. Life is dear because it holds a rich promise.

We find a positive attitude toward life in the Upanishads, in the Gita and in later literature. The world is the manifestation of the Divine. The Gita tells us that the Divine is working in the world, trying to shape it according to an idea. The man who has insight into this cosmic purpose, and expresses himself in harmony with it, lives a true life. The world is not without meaning but the meaning is not wholly contained therein.

A true life is a life in which action and contemplation blend. A life of contemplation without action is empty. We need both power and vision, strength and wisdom to make life meaningful. We need the experiences of the world in order to grow. There is nothing wrong with the world except our attitude toward it. Our individuality requires expression. The Gita asserts that nature cannot be suppressed. It is better to die following one's own nature than to imitate another's virtue. Truth has many levels. The different truths of our being need legitimate expression. Life should be honest and sincere.

It is the worldly attitude that is decried in the Upanishads — that outlook which makes the world, its success and pleasure, its power and glamor, our gods. The blind pursuit of such phantoms estranges men from their essential truth and lures them into greater bondage. There is a Sanskrit saying: "By unrighteousness men prosper, gain what they desire, and triumph over their enemies, but at the end they are destroyed at the roots."

Many find in sex and economics the meaning of life and reason of it all. The consequence of this is that the goal of life for many has become relief from tension. Aldous Huxley has remarked in one of his novels that the scourge of the Middle Ages was Black Death; the plague of the twentieth century is Grey Life. The "cultural" facilities of today are mostly distractions to keep younger people from mischief and older ones from emptiness. "Man drowns in the noise of the crowd his own clamor of silence."

In the Upanishads, life is pictured as a pilgrimage into the heart of the eternal. Life needs its legitimate expressions appropriate to the age and temper of the individual before it can ripen into the simplicity and purity of wisdom. Man's life is growth. He is a being in a state of transition. He has both the divine and the animal in him. There is nothing wrong with the animal as such; it is how the animal expresses itself which determines its value. The animal has to be given its due or it will not release us from its fetters. The animal may help or hinder our divine self-expression.

Commenting upon the story of the ancient fight between the gods and the titans mentioned in one of the Upanishads, an ancient interpreter remarks that the story is a mythical representation of the war that is being waged forever in the hearts of men between the forces of light and the powers of darkness. The forces of light are the impulses of life governed by spiritual insight and the powers of darkness are the same instincts self-centered and blind in their action. A true and meaningful life is one which has come to terms with all sides of the personality and become integrated on the basis of a spiritual insight. Repression brings suffering and hinders growth. But the repression from which civilized man suffers today is not the repression of the instincts, but of the divine in man.

YOGA AND ASCETICISM

It has often been thought that extreme asceticism and celibacy are the marks of a yogi and the conditions of Self-knowledge. This is not true. While there are ascetics and celibates who call themselves yogis, there are still other yogis who are not so.

The great teachers of the Upanishads, the founders of yoga, were family men who instructed their sons in Self-knowledge. A number of them were kings and rulers, active in debate and war. The two great teachers of Hinduism were Rama and Krishna, both of them princes and married men.

We are told in the Gita that the most fortunate birth for a person who aspires to be a yogi is to be born in the family of a yogi.

Hindu spiritual literature, the Vedas, the epics, the Puranas and the Tantras, is replete with accounts of men and women, highborn and outcasts, from all walks of life, who attained the highest knowledge of yoga through enlightened living, following their diverse occupations. The great Hindu epic, THE MAHABHARATA, of which the Gita forms a part, relates how a housewife and a hunter instructed a proud ascetic in higher wisdom.

Yoga is no retreat from the world; it is not a repressive but a directive psychology.

Monasticism is of comparatively late growth in India. While it has its reasons, the Gita, or the authentic yoga tradition, has not accorded it the highest honor.

Intelligent asceticism in the sense of self-discipline has a place in all spiritual life, in the formation of character. But extreme asceticism has been condemned as senseless and unspiritual by the Gita as well as by other books and teachers.

Celibacy may be adopted as a way of life by a few — I am not talking of celibacy late in life — if they so choose and are so fit by nature; if they want to avoid the troubles and cares of a family life which prevent concentration on spiritual exercises. In such a case, to be honest and true, they should live away from society as did celibates of ancient India. Also, in such an event, the society should support their simple life in return for their effort toward keeping spiritual values alive.

But these conditions are rarely met. Most of those who live in monasteries are not so spiritually equipped. Many are unfit for contemplation. They often live a quite comfortable life far above the level of the many humble people who support them. Some try to smother their troubled and guilty conscience with superficial excuses. No doubt members of many monasteries perform kind and useful social functions, but their individual lives are mostly lives of unprofitable constraint. Many have morbid feelings and attachments, indulge in food and drink, and can be quite cruel and vindictive, jealous and deceitful. Their minds are closed and their lives do not possess the vitality which might inspire men of strong individuality who love a richer life of freedom and experience and who do not care to play it safe as prisoners of an institution. Institutions and organizations may do a lot of good even though the individuals who compose them may lack real life. On the other hand, for the sake of religious institutions, members often do things which would make a truly kind man ashamed.

In the times of the Upanishads, persons who retired into the forest for contemplation did so after having lived a full life. They did not join an institution. They lived alone. They grew into the life of quiet contemplation naturally.

The Upanishads, however, decreed that the first quarter of the normal life of an individual, i.e. the first 25 years, was to be devoted to study, during which the student should observe celibacy. This regulation was for the Dvijatis. It is fitting that young people grow up in innocence. Good values, habits of self-control and self-discipline should be instilled into them by the teachers and parents who guide them. Without such discipline they will not be fit to make proper judgments in life. A mind undisciplined is like a body untrained; it will not stand up to the stresses and strains of living.

For nearly all men, a normal love life is an essential condition of growth into proper manhood and spirituality. Sex is neither wrong nor sinful; it is absurd to think so. It is the way we use it and look at it which makes it either good or bad. Sex is part of love. The act by which men live, by which love is expressed and by which the race is perpetuated, is not regarded as sinful by the Hindu. But we have a feeling of shame because sex is such a powerful drive that under its influence we often lose sense and self-control becoming selfish and mean, using other individuals as means to our end. It is normal for civilized consciousness to look upon weakness, lack of control and reason, as matters for shame and ridicule. Under the influence of sex, people often become forgetful of their obligations; they become blind and deceitful, dishonest and mean, ugly and vulgar, cruel and sordid—in a word, they become that incarnation of selfishness, the devil. They lose sight of the higher function and promise of life. It is for this reason people fear sex. A civilized person wants to have the strength and freedom to love. He wants to grow through love. But life is difficult and the ideal not easy to attain. It is enough if we try not to be blind. We cannot grow without mistakes; none is born perfect. If we shut the door to all error, we close the door to truth as well. No failure can stop us from finding truth; only the acceptance of failure can hide it from us.

We cannot love without character, nor can we have character without love. The Hindus believe that through love it is possible to realize perfection. They say: In the woman who is good, man feels Him; in the one who is true, man knows Him. India recognized long ago that woman is an inspiration to man, unconsciously guiding his restless energy into an immense variety of creation in literature, art, music and religion. She has therefore been called the Shakti, symbol of the creative power of the universe.

The eternal freedom of the soul can be found in love. People in love sometimes catch a fleeting glimpse of the noble and divine in man but, for lack of preparation and character, the vision dims and dies and life sinks once more to the level of the commonplace and insignificant.

Yoga is not the cessation of human relationships. It is the cessation of that bondage born of weakness. It is a new relationship through strength and freedom — a relationship that brings joy and not suffering. As long as we have not discovered our true Self our relationship with the world is imperfect and the cause of unhappiness.

YOGA AND PERSONALITY

Yoga is not the denial of true personality, but rejects the illusion of our separate individuality, our identification with the conditions of consciousness. To attain the emancipation of consciousness, the Universal or Cosmic Consciousness or whatever you may term it, we have to transcend the bounds of the changing conditions of nature, the flux of body and mind, the psychophysical processes which condition our individuality. The substantiality of ego is an illusion and, for that matter, the substantiality of anything is an illusion. Such notions of substantiality are the basis of our everyday life. We cannot be free unless we perceive their illusory character and regain our touch with reality.

When the illusory notions disappear nothing real vanishes with them. What we call the ego remains, but becomes related to the Impersonal beyond. Instead of being seen as our true Self, this newly balanced ego is seen as an instrument of the Self. To attain to this realization, we need the highest development of what we call our personality; the highest development that is, of reason and objectivity, and moral character.

It is ridiculous to say that yoga advocates suppression of individuality or regression to some plane of primeval mass consciousness. Can one think of a Rama, a Krishna, a Buddha, a Socrates, or in our own day of a Tagore or a Gandhi as lacking in personality, in freedom of mind and courage of heart?

We reach the essence of our being through the process of detachment and isolation, which is another name for giving up the wrong kind of relationship with nature. The process of life and progress of evolution is toward the isolation of consciousness from nature. It is a movement toward the freedom of consciousness. When, in the process of earth's evolution, a boulder became detached and distinct from a mountain mass it acquired a definite character which distinguished it from the rest, isolated it; it thus became some kind of an individual. Later, when plants came into existence, a higher type of individuality appeared. The plant, with its individual life, is more distinct from the inorganic environment than the boulder. Still later, animals came upon the scene and a further isolation from nature took place. The animal shares life processes with the plant but is not rooted in the natural environment. It has more freedom because it has the power of locomotion; it can range from place to place in its search for food, while the plant must draw its nourishment from the soil where it is rooted.

Man goes a step further in detaching himself from the environment. The animal has conciousness, but it is only a mass or herd conciousness; it is part of the animal world. Man has self-conciousness through which he isolates and distinguishes himself from other men. This, however, is not the end of evolution. Man grows through further differentiation and development of conciousness. Man evolves on the moral and rational plane as his identification shifts from the merely physical and vital to the ideal. The process of isolation and progressive release from the domination of nature is complete when man is no longer chained to his instincts, and consciousness is realized as distinct from the flow of thoughts and sensations. Then one knows one's true essence and the body and mind are seen as instruments of the Spirit.

YOGA AND SOCIETY

Another false notion which is widespread is that yoga philosophy and Hindu religion preach a kind of selfish self-absorption, ignoring one's duty and obligation to one's neighbor. In one word, yoga is considered other-worldly. A professor in a well-known university once remarked in a class on ethics that yoga advocates a moral holiday! A smart remark which sums up the point of view, but how absurd!

Some think that ethics form the essence of religion and that if a man looks beyond ethics, he is after illusions and disregardful of his obligation, neglectful of human concern and somehow out of touch with reality. However, in no other religious literature of the world do we find such a universal concern with society and humanity as in the Gita. Krishna, the teacher of the Gita, insists that Arjuna, his disciple and a prince, do his duty to king and country and not be deterred by any personal motive, however spiritual its manifestation. The Divine, the Gita declares, is active in the world at every moment, shaping its history. Man's activity should be in tune with this divine purpose. Man's life and progress depend on society, and a person who does not repay his debt to society with some form of service is like a thief.

We justify our existence by some kind of service. The feeling of obligation is planted deep in our heart. Many persons today are restless and guilt-laden because they feel they give nothing for what they receive.

The burden of the Gita's teaching is action with vision.

But the Gita is not a book of ethics alone. It is a spiritual scripture and teaches a higher obligation, obligation to truth. Society does not exhaust the significance of life. The meaning of life is ultimately to be found in Self-knowledge. Man does not find the answer to his striving or make sense of life until he actualizes the spiritual truth of his personality.

Whitehead once remarked that religion is what an individual does with his own solitariness. Society is not our goal. Those who make society their goal gradually reduce man to the insignificance of a robot or thing. Further, they, who do not see through the illusion of their narrow and separate individuality, end up in despair or disenchantment.

Social life and effort are meaningful. They help us to live, to grow and to reach our goal. Morality is the realization of unity in life through feeling and action; knowledge is the realization of the unity of existence through ideas and reflection. The justification of life's action lies in the attainment of wisdom and serenity of mind.

There will never come a time when society will be perfect and human suffering at an end. There will always be some who will suffer and others who will cause suffering. Nor will the world and society endure everlastingly. But our efforts must continue. Yoga alone makes sense of our feeling and effort. But for others, morality is no more than a matter of emotion lacking any higher justification in truth.

As early as the 4th century B.C., a great spiritual king of India, who gave up war and violence, built hospitals for men and animals — the first institutions of their kind in history. The great leaders of modern India have all drawn inspiration for their work from the Gita and the Upanishads. Gandhi worked politically because he wanted to find God through service to man, the yoga of action. Yoga is not aloofness from the world.

Nowhere else do we find so much absurd and morbid talk about devil and sin, flesh and spirit, vale of tears and vanity of vanities; such weeping and wailing, such whining and groaning about the world, such condemnation of the natural man and disparagement of worldly values, as in the literature of the Western religions.

The Upanishads and the Gita sanctify and hallow life and the world. Ignorance and prejudice, smugness and spiritual immaturity have combined to present the Hindu outlook on life as pessimistic and negative. There is also much propaganda advanced by those with unworthy motives. The popular superstitions and the curious practices of the ignorant masses are held up as Hinduism. I once heard a retired missionary in a university lecturing to graduate students on Hinduism. This was part of a general course, and I understood that the gentleman had taught the same subject for several consecutive years. He presented, with unconcealed glee, the bloody sacrifices and bizarre practices of some primitive Hindu communities as the quintessence of Hinduism. Somewhat like presenting the

Kentucky snake-cult as Christianity. Apparently he had never heard of the Upanishads or the Gita, or chose not to mention them. It is like lecturing on Christianty without knowing or mentioning the Bible.

There are others who know the Upanishads and the Gita but dismiss their teaching as "pantheism". If they find any social concern among Indian leaders or in Indian literature they immediately trace it to Christianity. The attitude is: Can anything good come out of Nazareth? One can only marvel at such blindness and smugness.

But there have been a number of men of perception who have felt the deep truth of Hinduism and who have recovered their faith in spiritual life through it. Scholars like Arnold Toynbee and others in our time are beginning to see that the western religions will have to be deepened and broadened by their contact with oriental thought if they are not to lose their hold on the minds of men liberated by science.

YOGA AND BUDDHISM

Earlier I have mentioned Hinduism in connection with Buddhism while speaking of yoga. People often wonder, what is the relation of yoga to Hinduism and Buddhism? Generally poor ideas exist on the subject.

Buddhism is commonly represented as different from Hinduism, and one sometimes gets the impression, while reading accounts by western writers, that it appeared on Indian soil like a bolt from the blue. Some consider Buddha's teaching as radically different from Hinduism and yoga. Buddhism is also characterized as a reform movement within Hinduism; somewhat like the Protestant movement within Christianity.

Buddhism is part of Hinduism. The Buddha was born a Hindu; he lived a Hindu and died a Hindu. He was one of the prophets and teachers of Hinduism. He is in line with the teachers of the Upanishads who preached a pure spiritual religion as opposed to the popular, priestly religion of heavenly life and sacrifices. All the basic categories of his thought as well as his terminology are taken from Hinduism. *Nirvana* (freedom), *prajna* (wisdom), *karma* (law of action) *avidya* (ignorance), *samadhi* (meditation), *samsara* (trans-migration) are all Hindu, pre-Buddhistic, terms and concepts. The ethics and the practice of meditation he taught are essentially those of yoga. His formulation of the four basic truths of existence, which he called the four *Aryan* (noble) truths, was traditional. The four basic truths are: (1) that there is suffering in the world, (2) that there is a cause for this suffering, (3) that there is an end to suffering, and (4) that there is a way to end suffering. Long before his time, Hindu medical books formulated the medical problem in the same manner. This fourfold classification of the problem of human suffering is also common to yoga.

In the Hindu tradition, spiritual philosophy is a kind of therapy for the cure of man's suffering (his ontological neurosis, if you so prefer and want to be modern and pedantic). The Buddha, in the tradition of the yogis, taught the way to end the disease of worldliness through the perception of truth.

A Professor of Religion once remarked facetiously to a class that Buddhism was the only good that India found exportable. This is a measure of popular ignorance on the subject. For one thing, Buddhism is part of Hinduism. For another, the teachings of the Upanishads and the Gita, quietly and without fanfare, have traveled and have been traveling beyond India's borders from pre-Buddhistic times. And further, other forms of Hinduism spread to many parts of Asia, providing inspiration to art, literature and music through the centuries.

The later *Mahayana* Buddhism with its doctrine of compassion and concern for the world, with its ideal of the *Amitabha* Buddha, the Buddha of limitless effulgence and compassion, is known as Sanskrit Buddhism. It started in India, and it is indebted to the Gita for its emphasis on action and its singular attitude to the world and man.

In a recent book, a teacher of philosophy who loves to draw distinctions, mentions Tagore time and again as a product of Hindu-

Buddhist thought, implying that Tagore got something from Buddhism which was not to be found in Hinduism. It is amazing. Tagore was brought up from childhood on upanishadic teachings and practice, on the literature and thought of the mystic poets of medieval India, especially those of Bengal. He no doubt worshipped Buddha, as every Indian does, as one of India's and the world's great prophets. He did so because he was a Hindu.

The Buddha made a great impact upon history mostly because of his unique personality which held in a rare combination so many excellences — supreme self-denial, mightly intellect, great heart, dominant will and limitless energy. However he is not the only Hindu whose message has been heard abroad. He did not claim to teach a new truth but, rather, the old perennial truths that had been taught through time by the earlier buddhas. Buddha means an enlightened person. Sri Krishna, the teacher of the Gita, spoke before the time of the Buddha in the same manner, teaching an ancient doctrine.

The Buddha is great not because he discovered a new idea or found a new way, but because he made the eternal truth of spirit dynamic and living through his experience and character. He brought the highest truth to the masses in their own language. His great intellect avoided all metaphysical nonsense; his great heart sought to remove all violence and false distinctions from society. He derided pretentions based on birth. He was intensely practical; his religion was simple and unencumbered.

The teachers of the Upanishads paid no attention to the artificial distinctions of birth and ancestry although they did demand fitness from students who sought their instruction. The Chhandogya Upanishad (c. 1200 B.C.) records the story of a young boy named Satyakama who approached a great teacher seeking instruction. The teacher as usual asked for references; wanted to know what family the boy came from and who his father was. The boy did not know. He said he had asked his mother but the mother had said she did not know. While she was young she had worked as a maid in many families and had conceived him during that time. She did not know who his father was. She told him that her name was Jabala, and his Satyakama; that he should introduce himself as Satyakama, son of Jabala. Upon listening to the story the teacher said, "Come my boy, I will initiate you; none other than a true Brahmin could speak out a truth so damaging to himself; you are born in the line of truth." Great teachers of India down to the present times have disregarded laws and conventions which do not embody truth.

YOGA AND HINDUISM

I now turn to the question of yoga and Hinduism. In the popular mind, Hinduism is a religion like Christianity or Mohammedanism and its distinguishing marks are caste, the sacred cow, vegetarianism and many gods, or some such nonsense.

It is not easy to give an idea of the depth and complexity of that which goes by the name of Hinduism. First of all, Hinduism has never been a religion in the sense in which the great religions of the world are understood. It was not founded by one leader, or a special line of prophets. It does not claim a precise historical origin. It does not have a set of well-defined beliefs based on the teachings of such founders, nor has it any special book which contains the most authoritative declaration of its principles and tenets. A religion is usually identified with a book, a prophet and a creed. Religion is a body of beliefs and practices centering round the idea of a divine personality who is the creator of nature and man, whose will has been revealed to the founder-prophet and whose commands must be obeyed by men in order that they be pleasing in his sight, acquire prosperity, or gain entrance to heaven. Hinduism is not a religion in this sense, though the concept of a divine ruler of nature and the hope of gaining heaven through good works are to be found in it. Hinduism is a complex phenomenon; it has both a social and a religious side. The substance of what goes by the name of Hinduism is formed by the teachings of the Vedas, the Upanishads, the Gita, the Puranas and other books. To put it succinctly, the Hindu believes that the Divine dwells in the heart of man and the ultimate fulfilment of life lies in the realization of this truth.

The vedic teachings came to be overlaid with the beliefs and practices of many peoples and cultures, primitive tribes, successive hordes of invaders, men of different races and tongues who settled in India and came to be integrated, with the passage of many centuries, into one very pluralistic society. Their many customs and beliefs found a philosophical basis in the spiritual doctrines of the Upanishads and the Gita. Many crude notions and practices died, many remained among people who were not cultivated enough. But all came to be informed by the spirit of the Gita and the Upanishads. The essential truth of religion sank deep into the consciousness and practice of the common masses. They came to look upon different religious views as different expressions of one truth. Above all they came to regard religion as experience and paid the highest respect to yogis or men who had attained spiritual wisdom. Followers of yoga appeared in all communities.

Hinduism is properly the name of a society and not a religion. The Hindus do not call their religion Hinduism; the different sects or groups who follow different disciplines according to their teachers call themselves and their faiths by different names. The word *Hindu* means Indian. It was first used by the Persians and the Greeks to denote the people of the Indus Valley or beyond, and is derived from *Sindhu,* which is the Sanskrit name for the river Indus. The Persians pronounced Sindhu as *Hindu,* while the Greeks made it into *Indus.*

The Hindus who derive their faith from the Vedas and Upanishads call it the *manava dharma* (the religion of man), *sanatana dharma* (perennial religion) or *arsha dharma* (the religion founded and revealed by the rishis, that is seers, or men of supersensuous experience). The revelations do not stop, nor do they come to men alone. Some of the greatest teachers have been women. Perception of truth is open to all at all times. Anyone can be a yogi. Yoga is the substance of Hinduism.

EAST AND WEST

I now bring this section to a close. My aim was to provide a perspective and to clear the atmosphere somewhat of the fog which fills it in order that things may be a little more lucid. However, to avoid any other kind of misunderstanding, I will end with a quotation from Tagore, taken from an essay written more than forty years ago:

"I have been fortunate in coming into close touch with individual men and women of the Western countries, and have felt with them their sorrows and shared their aspirations. I have known that they seek the same God—even those who deny Him. I feel certain that, if the great light of culture be extinct in Europe, our horizon in the East will mourn in darkness. It does not hurt my pride to acknowledge that in the present age Western humanity has received its mission to be the teacher of the world; that her science, through the mastery of the laws of nature, is to liberate human souls from the dark dungeon of matter. For this very reason I have realized all the more strongly, on the other hand, that the dominant collective idea in the Western countries is not creative... It is wholly wanting in spiritual power to blend and harmonize; it lacks the sense of the great personality of man.

"The most significant fact of modern days is this, that the West has met the East. Such a momentous meeting of humanity, in order to be fruitful, must have in its heart some great emotional idea, generous and creative. There can be no doubt that God's choice has fallen upon the knights-errant of the West for the service of the present age; arms and armour have been given to them; but have they yet realized in their hearts the single-minded loyalty to their cause which can resist all temptations of bribery from the devil? The world today is offered to the West. She will destroy it, if she does not use it for a great creation of man. The materials for such a creation are in the hands of science; but the creative genius is in man's spiritual ideal.

The limit to man's growth is his vision; there is no end to man's self-expression. Anything which helps the reality of man to emerge from the obscure depths of his personality is yoga, whether it comes from East or West.

II
PRINCIPLES

II

PRINCIPLES

YOGA AND THE YOGAS

The word *yoga* means both the perception of Self which is the goal, as well as the disciplines leading to it. The word literally means joining or harnessing the mind to Self. Yoga and yoke derive from a common root.

The direct means of perception is perfect concentration or calmness of mind. All means which help toward this realization are also yogas. Any form of discipline which helps to remove the veil of illusion and ignorance which obscures truth is yoga. The veil is our cocksure knowledge about the Self and the world. All feelings, thoughts and actions which contribute to the destruction of this illusion form part of yoga.

In the widest sense all life is yoga because the same secret urge for the manifestation of the truth lies behind all activity. But only a few people follow the goal intelligently and with vision, while others grope blindly in the dark. We are all seeking the same ideal, knowingly or unknowingly.

Yoga, is therefore both the means and the end, the road and the destination, the way and the goal.

In course of time, yogic practice came to be classified according to the place and importance a particular discipline occupied in the life of an individual. Thus arose the well-known divisions of yoga, namely, *Raja* Yoga, *Jnana* Yoga, *Bhakti* Yoga and *Karma* Yoga. These divisions make their first appearance in the epic poem, THE MAHA-BHARATA. They are clearly delineated in the Gita. In later books, we not only find mention of the four cardinal yogas but also of many subdivisions, e.g. *Mantra, Laya, Hatha,* and others.

Raja yoga literally means the royal yoga or the yoga *par excellence,* i.e. the yoga of concentration. This is a later designation. In earliest times it was called *Samkhya* yoga; *Samkhya* signifying the theoretical and yoga the practical aspect of the same discipline. *Jnana* yoga is the way of philosophical analysis and discrimination. *Karma* yoga is the way of action, while *Bhakti* yoga is the way of love and devotion.

The distinctions are mostly matters of emphasis. In actual practice the yogas are more or less mixed. Karma yoga suits men of vital, active and outgoing nature, but no action can be a yogic action unless it is informed by a spiritual attitude. The karma yoga of the Gita is blended with *jnana* (knowledge), *bhakti* (devotion) and *dhyana* (meditation). Men of a predominantly emotional nature are fit for the yoga of devotion. Men of intellectual and reflective nature incline to the yoga of philosophical analysis and contemplation. In the ideal yogi, like Krishna, there is an unusual richness of life and character due to a marvelous balance of reason, emotion and action.

Of the subdivisions of yoga, hatha yoga is the best known. Hatha yoga developed as a branch of raja or dhyana yoga. Yogis found out very early that suitable postures and regulated breathing were of great help in turning the mind inward. Hatha yoga grew out of this discovery. Later, other techniques were developed to gain extraordinary control over the body, to keep it strong, healthy and resistant to disease, decay and death.

Hatha literally means force or violence. The idea behind hatha yoga was to create the physical conditions for superconscious awareness. In the most heightened stage of concentration, the body becomes perfectly still; the physiological processes are almost completely arrested. This condition of the organism follows naturally and inevitably the state of *samadhi* or superconscious awareness. The hatha yogi's original aim was to create this condition by a long, complicated process of physical training, cleansing and fasting so that the mind could be more easily withdrawn and made perfectly calm.

In course of time, hatha yoga came to be developed in an extraordinary manner for the physical power and benefits it brought. Many who were attracted to it lacked high spiritual motive and understanding. The original rational outlook was overlaid in many cases with fancies and dogmas of various kinds. Divorced from its spiritual motive, it became an elaborate technique for gaining control over the body and its functions. Through long practice and devotion, some acquire a marvelous mastery over the body and preserve youthful health and vitality for a long time. They can do feats which astound people such as remaining buried under earth for several days, stopping heart-beats, swallowing poison, and making the body rigid like stone or steel. Neither spirituality nor consideration of health and vitality demand such practices. People who perform them are generally crude, lacking in perception and purity of motive. They dazzle others who come to think of yoga in terms of such abnormal power and contortionism. Sensationalism and exhibitionism are far removed from the true spirit and aim of yoga.

It is for such reasons that spiritual teachers came to look askance at the more extreme practices of hatha yoga. However, the simple principles and practices of hatha yoga are excellent for preserving youthfulness and health, improving body function and recovering lost powers. They improve posture and figure, retard aging and decay, relax tension and strengthen nerves. Combined with the practice of meditation, hatha yoga is, without a shade of doubt, the best form of physical culture and hygiene for the civilized man. The problem of health in a modern society, where people are somewhat free to choose their own values, is largely a problem of attitude. The correct practice of hatha yoga goes a long way toward solving this problem.

Today, the advance of medical knowledge makes possible a more intelligent application of hatha yoga principles.

The *mantra* and *laya* and other yogas are minor subdivisions of either bhakti or raja yoga. *Mantra* means a word, syllable or phrase with sacred associations. Mantra yoga is repetition of such syllables or words with meditation on their meanings. Such repetitions (preferably silent and inward) are useful for many beginners in spiritual practice. Rosary and repetition of names began in India. The practice was adopted by other countries and later incorporated into many religions, including Greek Orthodoxy, Roman Catholicism and Sufism.

Laya means merging i.e. merging the mind in the Self through concentration on a sound or idea. It is only a variation of raja yoga. There are other minor variations and subdivisions of yoga which arose to suit individuals of different temperament. These forms of discipline were developed and continue to be practiced by various groups and sects. However, the necessary thing to have is a grasp of the basic, universal principles and practices of yoga. But first it is important to consider the question of power which has been raised by our discussion.

YOGA AND POWER

Yoga is both knowledge and power. The search for knowledge is closely related to the search for power. "Knowledge is power" is an ancient Sanskrit saying. Francis Bacon also made the same remark.

The power which a yogi seeks is the power that destroys basic or philosophical ignorance. This power is the knowledge or realization of our true nature. Such knowledge liberates us from those delusions which are the cause of our weakness and suffering. However, through certain yogic practices special powers of perception as well as power over natural forces and things come to us. These powers are not without limit, nor are they ever-lasting. Yoga regards the pursuit of such powers as unspiritual, as creating further bondage and leading, ultimately, to suffering.

The people who pursue power for selfish personal ends are materialists. The powers they gain are not secure. Selfish use of power destroys the clarity of mind and detachment which made their acquisition possible, thus leading to their ultimate loss. Pursuit of those ends which run counter to the march of life and the universal concerns of history comes to grief sooner or later.

In the affairs of the world, men often gain power through service to interests larger than their own. As long as power truly serves, it is secure. But the moment power becomes corrupt, which happens more easily than might be supposed, it nurses fear, invites attack and so moves ultimately towards its own downfall.

Napoleon's ambition coincided for a time with the liberating forces of democracy and nationalism. He was swept on their tides to heights of success and glory. But when he lost touch with the historic trends and tried to feed his personal ambition, he only succeeded in bringing about his own ruin.

The same law operates in the field of higher yogic power. The interest in power is natural. But preoccupation with power prevents growth and deflects us from the true goal.

Intelligent people recognize the limitation of material power while others are so confused that they forget the most basic and natural satisfactions of life. Intoxicated with power and success, they seek them as ends in themselves. The consequences are much too evident around us. Many people achieve material success fairly early in life, but the very means which enable them to achieve their fortunes render them incapable of enjoying their prize. The mad race toward power is paid for in ulcers and heart conditions; life is filled with tension and framed by anxiety. Such people live without love or peace and spend most of their days under the care of doctors, psychiatrists and lawyers.

Misconception about power is all the more unfortunate in the case of those who seek spiritual freedom.

SAMADHI OR SUPERCONSCIOUS EXPERIENCE

Samadhi or superconscious experience is the key concept of yoga. Yoga as philosophy is an interpretation of existence based on this experience; it is life viewed in the perspective of *prajna,* or truth-filled wisdom, and the estimation and organization of values in that perspective. It is also a method for the progressive realization of man's supreme goal of truth. It is therefore essential to have an understanding of samadhi, its relationship to life and to the evolution of man.

All religions are ultimately based on experience of the beyond. A religion, as a creed, is not truth; it is only a way. People need creeds and beliefs to organize their lives and give them sensible direction; society needs institutions to preserve ideals and to guide men. But beliefs and institutions are not the resting places of the mind. It has been said: It is good to be born in a church but terrible to die in it. Beliefs are provisional, they acquire fresh meaning with experience. Besides, men do not know the meanings of their beliefs. God, heaven, and salvation mean different things to different individuals at different levels of development. No one has clear ideas about them.

Real religion begins with experience. The test of a true religious experience is seen in the transformation of character and in the achievement of a clearer comprehension of the realities of existence.

When we come to the realm of religious experience we encounter many varieties which depend on the training and background of the individual involved. There is an infinite range. But as we move higher and higher into more universal areas, the differences in expression lessen and finally disappear. In the experience of pure Awareness, the distinction between knower and known is lost. One who achieves the experience exclaims, 'I am the Truth', 'I am Brahman', 'Thy Self is Brahman'. This is the experience of the pure Selfhood and is the highest form of samadhi, or superconsciousness. In yoga this is technically called *nirvikalpa* samadhi, or *asamprajnata* samadhi.

Superconsciousness has also been called cosmic or universal

consciousness. In this state the limitations of consciousness, spirit or pure Self, fall away. One discovers one's true identity as transcendent spirit and clearly perceives the basic unity of existence. Samadhi is the height of awareness and the essence of yoga; it is the perfect apprehension of Truth and the supreme achievement of man, his highest value. Yoga is also called samadhi. The Gita says:

> Gaining which man does not consider any other gain superior,
> And established in which he is not shaken by the greatest pain,
> Know that state above suffering to be yoga...

Some theologians have made a great fanfare about the superior value of dogmatic faith and the dualistic religious attitude based upon it. They regard mystic experience as subjective, personal and without social significance, maintaining that the relation of "I and Thou" is a more objective relationship which invests individual life and world history with meaning and worth. We have seen earlier that yoga assigns a superior value and deeper significance to the everyday concepts of personality and social activity. It accepts the distinction between subject and object on the practical plane. But, philosophically and scientifically speaking, the distinctions are superficial and not radical, i.e. they are not ultimately true or valid. People work intellectually with such distinctions; they are dogmas and creeds. As creeds they have their value and also their limitations. But if they are not seen in their proper light, they bar man's growth and lead to fanaticism, with all the evils which come in its train. Subject and object are two phases of the same spirit. What we generally call subject is actually an object, the psycho-physical complex, our apparent self and identity. The pure subject as awareness is opposed to nature, as light is to darkness. In nirvikalpa samadhi we have the experience of the pure unconditioned Selfhood or subject. Nature or object is an emanation of the pure subject.

The lower form of samadhi or superconscious experience is called *savikalpa* samadhi or *samprajnata* samadhi, i.e. cognitive samadhi. On this plane the mind knows objects with a degree of concentration which is called *ekagra* and which is extraordinary. Such concentration reveals the subtle or finer truths of nature, the underlying principles of things.

The superior samadhi, i.e. the nirvikalpa samadhi is also called the *nirodha* samadhi or the perfect arrest of all forms of mental functioning. Patanjali defines yoga in this manner.

YOGA, EXISTENTIALISM AND ZEN

The mystery of creation is like the darkness of night—it is great.
Delusions of knowledge are like the fog of the morning.

This brings me to consider briefly another type of *I-Thou* relationship of which some modern theologians, known as existentialists, speak and which they distinguish from the I-It or the non-personal practical relationship of everyday life. However, it is significant to recall that ideas of the same kind, in a non-theological sense, are being advanced by many modern psychologists and thinkers who do not purport to be existentialists. They note and regret the almost exclusively marketing and exploitative orientation of modern life and the lack of genuine human relationship beyond the purely practical. Moving away from the narrow and individualistic categories of modern psychology these thinkers are beginning to recognize that man's freedom and fulfilment lie in the realization of his power to love and his selfless concern for fellow men.

This has drawn the attention of many in the West to yoga and zen, and there is a growing awareness today that existentialism, yoga and zen have something in common which is significant for the health and happiness of modern man who is asking questions about the meaning of life, but who cannot be satisfied by the dogmatic and authoritarian faiths of old. It is therefore appropriate that we pay a little attention to them in order to see what they have in common and where they part company.

Existentialism as a dominant trend of our time is not something novel in essence, but derives its meaning and importance from the context in which it has arisen. It reunites faith and philosophy, the bonds between which remained sundered for centuries, and it marks the beginning of a new era of general thought and attitude. Existentialism has destroyed for all time the pretensions of reason to understand existence in terms of clearcut formulas of intellect, and it has shattered the dream of science to turn the world into a paradise through control and comprehension of nature. Existentialism, further, has pointed up the remoteness of academic philosophies from life, the frivolity of much philosophic discussion and the endless, trite and inconclusive efforts over centuries to establish standards of goodness, beauty and truth.

Existentialism focuses attention on the concrete human situation and the central problems of existence. It brings to the fore the universal facts of death and anxiety which weigh upon the finite life of man. It speaks of the radicalness of evil and calls upon man to realize an authentic existence of his own through choice and action, through faith and dedication in a world which is uncertain and lacking in any special direction of its own.

If the god of old faith is dead, so also is the new goddess, Reason. We live in an age, neither of unchallengeable faith nor of cocksure reason.

Existentialism is however no denial of the function of reason, nor does it repudiate the need for a faith of some sort. After reason has done its best and found its own limits, thoughtful people stand as it were on the brink of the vast and deep mystery of Being. The awareness of the profundity of Being and its richness is a challenge; it is a call to openness of life and conduct.

Lacking any sure rational guide to our conduct, we are thrown back upon some kind of deliberate faith to explore the meaning of life through appropriate choice and action. The two broad wings of existentialism mention two alternatives for choice: faith in humanity or faith in God. This faith, whether theistic or atheistic, is not arbitrary and dogmatic in the sense in which the traditional faith is. Further it is a faith that attaches meaning to a life that transcends a purely egocentric and individualistic existence. Though, like so many other things, it cannot be rationally justified yet it offers reasons, existential reasons, for its choice. Moreover it is a faith which is open and which embraces the total personality of man. This act of faith is a leap in the dark in order to wrest some meaning from life which is otherwise tragic and absurd.

Such faith however is not untouched by either doubt or uncertainty, though the existentialist theologians do speak of the religious experience of the man of faith, which comes to him through grace and which transports him to a new dimension of authentic and meaningful existence above and beyond the ordinary — into a life of true and meaningful relationship with the world. Yet doubt and obscurities remain and the vision fades.

In a way, existentialism harks back to the old concept of philosophy as a way of life supported by critical thought. Philosophy is action; it is the active search for wisdom and truth of life, which is different from abstract intellectualism or pure scientism or the so-called scientific philosophy.

It will have been obvious that yoga is existentialist not only because it starts from the concrete human situation of man's finiteness and the problems attendant upon it but also for the reason that it is philosophy as practice which is nourished by rational thought. It is the search for and realization of the meaning of life and the truth of existence through action and contemplation. But it is also more, for it both includes and transcends faith and reason. It does not stop at a faith which is a leap in the dark, nor in an experience which is fugitive and uncertain.

Yoga presses forward beyond the existentialist attitude which is no final resting place of the mind. It develops subtle powers of perception beyond reason and simple faith. Its final achievement is samadhi or prajna, the Knowledge that is not knowledge, the purest awareness beyond all duality and relationship, the perfect unity of existence. To find truth we must become one with it in the supreme silence of contemplation. When through samadhi man experiences the unity underlying the skin-deep plurality of forms then, in the words of the Upanishads, the knots of his heart are sundered, all his doubts vanish and bondage to action ceases. After experience of samadhi, man's relationship with the world is transformed for good and he is no longer deluded and deceived by appearances. *"He whose self is united with Spirit by the practice of yoga sees the Spirit in all beings and all beings in the Spirit; he sees the same everywhere."* (The Gita.)

The Truth that makes one free is impersonal; that Truth is God. Man is not free until he transcends the limits of egoistic consciousness. The mystery of Truth is never communicated in language, nor do its expressions have any limit. The eternal surprises of the Infinite are inexhaustible. *"The Spirit is infinite; manifestation is infinite. The infinite emanates from the Infinite. Taking the infinite from the Infinite the Infinite remains."* (The Upanishad.)

Yoga affirms, as existentialism does, but much more radically, that man makes his own fate by his thought and action, choice and participation, by his karma. Man is free to choose freedom or bondage. But unlike some existentialists, yoga proclaims the essential divinity of man which will one day or other become manifest in all. Man can never be eternally lost; the spirit's urge for self-expression is continually pressing upon him to choose freedom through knowledge. Man is not an empty shell but holds divinity within him.

The more I read and hear of the *I-Thou* relationship, the more I feel that it is a form of romanticism far removed from the integral perception of truth. We need much more than the kind of faith of which it speaks to satisfy the spirit of man. Yoga begins with faith but goes beyond it. True faith ripens into indubitable experience.

> *"Faith is the bird that feels the light*
> *And sings when the dawn is dark."*

Yoga is the bright light of morning after the dawn of faith. It is puerile to talk of the mystic's attitude as rejection of life and world. Mysticism is rejection of illusions—the fundamental illusion of the radical separateness and plurality of things. Mystics reject the claim of the show to be the substance. They affirm the right attitude toward life and world. Is it not true, as it has been said in India, that they who scorn life raise life above scorn and that they who worship it make it mean? Life is paradoxical; its affirmation is also its rejection.

Truth, like life, is paradoxical. The supreme paradox of all is the extreme polarity of existence, the world of duality and change opposed to the realm of the One and Eternal.

A lot of confusion also exists regarding zen and its relationship to yoga. A few authors writing on zen present it as a unique phenomenon and as quite distinct from yoga, which they pronounce to be impractical and otherworldly. Zen is an abbreviation of the word *za-zen*, which is a Japanese version of the Chinese word *chan*, which again is Chinese for the yoga technical term *dhyana*, or contemplation. Zen is a particular school of Buddhism which has specially developed in Japan but it came by way of China, which received it originally in the sixth century from an Indian saint named Bodhidharma. Zen is derived from the teachings of the Buddha.

The zen school of Buddhism is a meditative school. Though it is characterized by some special techniques and methods, its essence is the essence of Buddhism. Zen arose as a protest against the intellectuals who became unduly preoccupied with futile logic-chopping and abstract philosophical speculations and forgot that ultrarational illumination which is the goal of Buddhism cannot be attained by rational thought but only by a shift of awareness beyond the ordinary levels of consciousness. Satori or enlightenment is the soul of zen; satori is prajna, satori is samadhi. Satori, nirvana, prajna and samadhi mean the same experience. The peculiar ceremonies, methods and attitudes of the zen school make it a distinct branch of integral yoga but not something essentially novel. In the vast orchestra of yoga, zen takes the place of a special instrument.

Zen has to be understood in the context of Mahayana Buddhism in which love and active service play a dominant role. People often forget this, and also the fact that zen presupposes arduous preparation for satori. The spontaneity and naturalness, the freedom from rites and ceremonies, from forms and rules, of which zen speaks have been emphasized by all men of profound spiritual perception as marks of true enlightenment. But such spontaneity and naturalness, freedom and joyous existence come after a long preparation and discipline.

There is a school of yoga in Bengal called the *Bauls* or madcaps who derive their religion from an ageless tradition. They call their way of life *sahaja*, that is, simple or natural. Nothing can surpass them in their rejection of forms and ceremonies, temples and creeds, rules and customs, books and laws, institutions and establishments, and in their emphasis upon the spontaneity and naturalness of life. They say, in the words of Kabir, the medieval saint of India:

> *I close not my eyes, nor torment my body.*
> *But every path I then traverse becomes a path of*
> *   pilgrimage to the Divine,*
> *Whatever work I do becomes service.*
> *This simple consummation is the best.*

The spontaneity of a great artist comes after long and arduous preparation; the suprarational beyond reason is not the irrational below it. The ultraviolet and the infrared rays are both dark to ordinary perception, but they dwell on opposite poles.

The special zen techniques for self-forgetful concentration, absorption, and non-verbal superior awareness do not make it a new spiritual phenomenon. There are myriad varieties of spiritual exercises that lead different kinds of aspirants to the same goal. The positive approach to life, the concreteness of spiritual experience, the divine awareness all the time rather than in rare moments of inward self-absorption, the communication of the higher truths of spirit through art—these are not the special property of any particular sect. One finds them often in the vast spiritual tradition of India.

MIND AND THE FORMS OF AWARENESS

The functions of the mind can be classified according to different principles. For example, we say that the mind can function not only on the conscious and preconscious planes, but also on the superconscious level. On this last level, the ordinary functions of the mind are completely arrested by the power of voluntary concentration. The feeling of "I" or the ego disappears on this plane and a person becomes established in his true being. He is no longer identified with the fluctuating states of the body or mind but discovers that his true nature is distinct from them. This superconscious state is the direct opposite of the egoless preconscious condition.

According to one system, the superconscious state has been described as a fourth state of awareness (*turiya*), distinguishing it from the states of deep sleep, dream and wakefulness. Still another view (as in Patanjali), differentiates pure awareness from five other forms of common mental function: right cognition (*pramana*), error (*viparyaya*), intellectual construction (*vikalpa*), memory (*smriti*), and sleep (*nidra*).

The last form of classification makes certain things clear. Superconscious knowledge, called prajna, is different not only from error, illusion, hypnotic trance, etc., but also from *right* knowledge, i.e. valid perceptions, inferences or communications. Thus it is different from "science" and "scientific" knowledge. Yogic knowledge, wisdom or perception is superior to the conceptual knowledge of science. Philosophical truth, in the sense of superconscious perception, is higher than scientific truth which is practically valid but not metaphysically true.

Vikalpa is a special type of mental function which deserves some comment since it has been generally misunderstood and mistranslated. *Vikalpa* designates empty concepts or intellectual constructs, i.e. those which have no objective counterpart but are nevertheless useful and to be found in all linguistic formulations. Such constructions are necessary for communication and practical, but they are no more than imaginings. Time and space, substance and quality are such notions. They are useful but unreal. There can be no language or statement without vikalpa. Linguistic truth is a relative truth. The "brute and stubborn facts" are burdened with a lot of wooly fiction.

Superconscious experience is the most immediate form of knowledge. This is the real intuitive knowledge of yoga. Such intuition is superior to reason, as reason is superior to the senses.

The perfect stillness of mind which is samadhi, is comparable to the smooth surface of a clear lake in which an object is mirrored perfectly without being broken up and distorted by waves. In an analogous manner, we perceive the clear reflection of the Self in the calm lake of the mind. Then we know our real Self (atman) in its pristine purity, for at all other times we are identified with the processes of the body and the mind.

The state of samadhi or perfect inwardness is achieved through the practice of concentration (abhyasa) and discrimination (vairagya), or detachment.

CONCENTRATION AND SAMADHI

The power of concentration is inherent in all minds. Perfect concentration or absorption of mind in an object, idea or emotion is not unknown to men in general. The mind according to yoga functions on five levels, at each of which a type of samadhi occurs. But samadhi on the first three of these levels is not the yogic samadhi, for it is without control and clarity.

The five levels of the mind are, 1) the infatuate or dull (mudha), 2) the passionate or|restless(kshipta),|3) the scattered or normal (vikshipta), 4) the one-pointed or concentrated (ekagra) and 5) the arrested or perfectly still (niruddha). On the infatuate or dull level the attention sometimes becomes so completely fixed on an object that the mind and the body cease to function. We describe this condition by such phrases as "numbed with pain" or "petrified with fear." On the second or passionate level the mind can also be completely absorbed in an object leading to a paralysis of mental and physical activity. Men are known to have died of heart failure under the influence of passion. But these concentrations are involuntary and are not yogic. It is on the third level of mind, i.e. the normal level that we find the exercise of rational control and the beginning of true concentration. Still, concentration is far from perfect on this plane. The mind continues to be incessantly swayed and drawn in many directions. It is restless like the wind.

The real yogic concentration occurs only on the fourth and fifth levels. When all the mental energy is fully focused on one object through conscious voluntary effort, we have samadhi on the ekagra, or one-pointed, level of mind. Such concentration is rare and supernormal and comes after long and steady practice. The subtle realities (tattvas) of nature are revealed in this samadhi. The ekagra samadhi has several stages according to its duration and its objects.

The last level is the plane of the arrested mind. At this point there is no object to occupy the mind which is perfectly still. This is the nirodha samadhi mentioned before, in which the Self which is pure Consciousness stands revealed without any modification or limitation.

YOGA AS AWAKENING

Yoga is the process of deconditioning the Self. It can also be described as a process of dehypnotization. Mankind lives in a general condition of hypnosis or make-believe. We take ourselves for what we are not and we take things around us for what they only seem to be. We project traits, conditions and qualities upon Self and nature where they do not belong. Eternal purity and freedom belong to Self essentially. It is illusion which creates fear and bondage—a hypnotic conditon. We are asleep on the plane of the spirit. That is why samadhi is called Awakening.

The yoga practices are for the sake of samadhi; they are steps leading to it. Spiritual disciplines are for the purification of the mind.

Purity of mind is clarity and calm, lucidity and objectivity. An impure mind is either dull or restless. It is a mind which is either torpid, immobilized by a preoccupation or helplessly active under irrational drives. Yoga practices bring the mind under control through conquest and integration. *"The mind is under the control of a yogi, a yogi is not under the control of mind."*

Yogic discipline brings into view and controls the unconscious mind and its sunken tendencies (*samskaras*). Thus the mind becomes truly integrated and dynamic.

LIFE AND EVOLUTION

Before turning to a discussion of the yogic disciplines, it will be meaningful to consider samadhi in relation to life and human evolution.

The central idea in life, evolution, civilization, and in science is the same: control and comprehension. It is conquest of self and nature through understanding. The dynamic principle behind the evolution of nature is the urge, secret and concealed, for the emancipation of consciousness from its subjection to matter. This is spiritual freedom. All other freedoms are means to this end—social, political and economic. An ideal society or community is one in which every member has all these necessary freedoms to grow into the fullest manhood, to come into his own. Whether such a society can be realized or not is another question, but that is the ideal which inspires men to action.

Man today stands on the highest plane of evolution. But evolution has not come to an end with the appearance of the self-conscious individual. The egoistic man is not the grand finale of evolution. Attainment of self-consciousness has been an essential gain for life but if that self-consciousness is to remain mere egotism and stubborn individualism, man will never realize his full development in spiritual freedom nor emancipate his consciousness from the illusion of the plurality and separateness of things. The whole drive of civilization is against false discrimination and toward the effectuation of the basic unity and solidarity of life. This is the goal as well as the justification of reason and morality. When the veil of illusory separateness of things is removed the fleeting forms of the world do not disappear but come together in the awareness of eternal Being which is the ineffable beauty spoken of in the Upanishads and by Plato.

Nature evolves for the freedom of man through experience. Man grows through his experience into understanding. His happiness lies in his sense of a meaningful journey to some real goal. In such a journey no experience is without some sense. The spirit's desire for emancipation is the motor of history. Yogis believe that there will come a time when all individuals without exception will fully realize the Divine potentiality in their lives. They will attain this state, whether it be called wisdom, jnana, prajna, satori, nirvana or cosmic consciousness. The few individuals, both men and women, who have so far attained this freedom, are the forerunners, the antennae of the race. These men, prophets and seers, appear like sudden mutations in the field of evolution. They have had revelations and intimations of spirit in different degrees. They indicate the future of man. They are the pathmakers (*pathikrit*). They call men to their immortal heritage.

Spiritual freedom has been the ever-present preoccupation of the self-conscious individual from the early dawn of civilization. The quest has taken many guises; the answer has appeared in different forms. Mostly it has come in the form of a faith or a religion. Religions contain the kernel of essential truth overlaid with a heap of fancies and myths. While offering hope, they have often created artificial divisions between life here and a life beyond, between nature and supernature. They have too often put feelings of irrational fear and guilt into the hearts of men by condemning the natural life and standing in the way of truth and reason, of humanism and self-expression. For this reason, many sensible people have turned away from religion in every age. Especially in our time, with the advance of science, the picture of God, world, and man as given in the popular religions appears ridiculous to thoughtful individuals. But the spiritual problem and the quest for freedom remain despite the decline and disappearance of many religious ideas and attitudes. Many have sought to deny or ridicule the spiritual problem as meaningless from lack of a deep understanding or want of philosophical competence. They are more or less bound by uncritical materialistic assumptions. Despite their rationality and insight in limited areas of life, they are without the experience and detachment necessary to view life objectively, as a whole.

Religion's continuing hold on millions of people shows that it is still instinctively felt that religion stands witness to the existence of something true and noble beyond the grasp of reason. And this, despite the fact that many of its dogmas are hardly worthy of belief.

The undying spiritual problem of man, the question of meaning in life, is appearing in the field of practical psychology and psychotherapy. The kind of problems which adults bring nowadays to many therapists and analysts are not the usual simple neurotic symptoms which can be cleared up by traditional techniques and formulas in a number of sittings. Modern man already knows much too much about inhibitions and repressions. The repression from which modern man suffers is not so much the repression of his instincts as the repression of the Divine in him. The problem is essentially one of recognizing the spiritual need and of finding some faith which can give meaning to life.

Psychology is becoming philosophical in a deeper sense. Many who deal with the problems of tension and anxiety are realizing the limitation of formulas evolved in an individualistic and materialistic framework for the comprehension and cure of such afflictions. Life is much too complex for such simple explanations. Psychotherapists are today confronting the basic problem of meaning in life, of freedom and humanity, as distinct from the troubles which arise from ordinary conflicts and repressions. Integration and individuation are no answer to the general neurosis of our time. Truly human problems emerge after such integration and individuation. The need is widely and increasingly being felt for a new outlook on life, for a faith that makes sense, a faith based not on materialistic, psychological or religious illusions, but on the deeper realities of existence, a faith adequate to the demands of the total human being.

It is a paradox, but faith in spirit brings hope to life and makes it truly creative. Reason without faith produces only despair, makes ethics a matter of taste, and man an alien in the universe. The "Freeman's Worship" is a whistle in the dark. True faith is not authoritarian, it is the fulfillment of reason. Truth can be achieved here and now. Samadhi is not an unobtainable goal.

Faith (bhakti) was defined by Shankara, the Indian philosopher-saint, as faith in one's Self. It is faith in Man. There is more in man than is suspected by many who talk of humanism. The test of a true philosophy lies in the strength and freedom, energy and inspiration it gives to an individual. The faith, which in practice enriches life, opens the heart and frees the mind from prejudice, fear and illusion, cannot but be true.

PURPOSE IN LIFE

Many who have become familiar with oriental philosophy, are confused in regard to some of its cardinal concepts and goals. One such difficulty has arisen in connection with the meaning of life and the nature of freedom. Some write as though yoga were no more than a form of psychotherapy, and freedom (moksha or nirvana) only a kind of intellectual wisdom and psychological integration. It is idle, they contend, to speak of life's meaning and vain to seek deep purpose in it since, according to both science and oriental thought, there is no individual as a substantive entity, the ego being an illusion; that people in the West, under cultural suggestions, worry themselves into needless anxiety and neurosis by asking such pointless questions. People should just recognize the scientific truth about the flux of things and patterns of processes, come to terms with the subconscious, and live without worry.

The Scottish philosopher Hume gave a classic expression to the fact that our ordinary perception reveals nothing but the unsubstantial character of what we call self. In ancient India there was a school of philosophical materialists, the *charvakas,* the first such school in history, which denied the reality of anything beyond the changing processes perceptible to the senses. They recommended a carefree life *a la Rubaiyat-i-Omar Khayyam,* without fussing over soul and salvation.

But things are not so simple. People continue to ask questions about life despite such prescriptions. They can't help it. They continue to believe that there is more than they see with their eyes.

Life is a difficult road to travel. We need understanding and guidance for our journey.

The ego, or the little self, has no substantiality and no ultimate significance; there is no goal, no resting place in the world, only transitory states. This perception, which is intellectual, may be the beginning of a spiritual query. But it is not the final wisdom of life. There is a larger life beyond the little self. In that context, the ego is not a meaningless appearance. To seek purpose in life is to strive to feel the positive Truth beyond which makes the illusion of ego possible and which inspires men to transcend the little existence we call our own.

People seek purpose in life. Life is not a mechanical movement. Thoughtful persons try to understand it in terms of its basic drives and goals. Unless we have some conception of our goals and take due cognizance of them, we run into trouble. Psychologists try to unify life's drives under some common principles, calling them libido, hunger, power, pleasure, love, understanding, etc. Others say that man seeks happiness. The question is what it is, how to find it, and by what means?

Those who do not see a supreme goal in life beyond the fulfillment of instinctual drives, or who see nothing beyond the limited meanings of individualistic existence, create all the serious problems of life.

All philosophy tries to see life as a whole rather than piecemeal. Life's supreme achievement lies in knowledge and understanding. This knowledge is integral; it is a perception.

We cease to ask these questions about life when we rise above the plane of intellect and the illusory ego sense. Then we are really free. But this freedom is not an intellectual idea, a negative concept. It is a positive state within the person achieved through meta-psychological perception.

Shankara states, in his introduction to the commentary on the *Brahma Sutras,* that from the standpoint of wisdom there is not much difference between the conduct of a man learned in philosophical doctrine and that of an animal. Both are governed by fear and passion. They are not free.

Only free men do not seek goals. They take delight in the Self *(atmarati);* they are established in themselves *(atmastha.)* Their life flows at ease, like leaves blown by the autumn winds. But this is not the case with those who have the pseudo-wisdom of science and intellect. Those who try to live from moment to moment, without any understanding of the direction and evolution of life and without the sense of a career, live at best uninspired lives. When they preach this wisdom to others they are, in the words of the Katha Upanishad, like the blind leading the blind.

TRUTH AND ILLUSION

I have spoken of truth and illusion in the preceding pages. It is therefore proper that I further clarify the meanings of these words and point out what they stand for in yoga philosophy.

Truth can be both perceptual *(aparoksha)* and conceptual *(paroksha).* Truth is both a fact and the quality of a statement. When yoga speaks of truth it means the ultimate or underlying fact of existence, the reality, or spirit. The experience which is ultimate and which is never contradicted by any other experience is the highest truth. This is the truth attainable by samadhi. Perception of truth shows up the illusory character of other experiences prior to it; therefore it is called prajna, the supreme knowledge, or wisdom. Knowledge here is not a theory or an abstract conception but a perception.

But there are levels of truth. First, there is truth on the rational and sense level. We lead our daily lives on this level. We know that what is presented to us by the senses is an appearance. There is something behind such appearances. Our reason gives us many theories in regard to the underlying facts and operations of nature. But they are never final. We have come to realize through rational investigation that in the very act of sensory observation we change and distort what we observe. We do not see or know the fundamental truth of things. The mystery remains and deepens and the usual notions, with which we carry on our practical life, are seen to be illusions. This awareness removes many prejudices and false beliefs, but is not important enough to give us true freedom.

There is another kind of illusion which surrounds our life until we wake up. It is the poor understanding of our selves, our nature and destiny. We live and act on the belief that we are individuals, but we do not know what this individuality is. We do not know what we really want. Today we may want one thing, tomorrow it is not enough for us, though we thought that if only we had it we would be happy all our life. Tastes and ideals change. Nothing is good for all time. The child's optimism gives away with the years to a sense of despair and disillusionment.

Recently (early in 1963) Bertrand Russell was interviewed for TV on the occasion of his ninetieth birthday. Asked to discuss the happiest period in his life, Russell replied that he had never been happier than he was at the moment. When the interviewer asked the reason, the philosopher replied that he now knew exactly what he wanted in life. If Bertrand Russell, with all his logic and clarity of mind, came to know at the age of ninety that the real meaning of his life lay in a humanistic concern transcending the limits and needs of his own individualistic existence, how much perception can be expected of others?

People do not realize the roots of their motivations and desires. They say they make conscious choices and decisions in life without realizing how much they are governed by unconscious universal forces. Under the influence of rage and passion, they often do things which they regret the rest of their lives. Seeking happiness by wrong means, they destroy the very conditions of happiness. A man who cannot respect himself, cannot be happy; he who rules others by fear cannot, himself be free from fear and anxiety. People who value power find that power, once achieved, does not satisfy the needs of the heart. Men cannot gain true love, affection, honor and respect by means of power.

Men are not fully awake. They like to live in dreams. They like to be told lies, to be told that they are loved and respected though in their hearts they know it is not so. This is what most people call life. They are so dependent, so helplessly alone, yet what an ego they have! One moment they shout and bluster, the next they weep and go down on their knees. A little praise and adulation transports them to the heavens; a little criticism and rebuke drives them to tears.

People do not live their lives, they are lived by it. They want to enjoy, they are enjoyed; they go out to catch, they get caught; they try to deceive, they are, themselves deceived; they want to be clever and prove themselves stupid.

Sensible persons realize late in life how they should have lived, but the time has already passed by.

Blindness about life and its goal is *avidya* or ignorance. *Avidya* is philosophical or metaphysical ignorance; basically, it is a false view of our Self, our true nature. Radical ignorance is shown in clinging to the notion of separate egohood and individuality, in regarding the impermanent as permanent, in identifying the process with reality. Because of this ignorance, man seeks peace, happiness and self-fulfillment through pursuit of worldly goods, pleasures, success and power.

Avidya is also called *Maya*. Avidya is a false view and not total ignorance. We live in a twilight zone, not in 'total darkness. Maya is no denial of plurality and change. But the world needs to be seen in the context of the Cosmos, the individual in the context of the universal, the person in the context of the impersonal, the many in the context of the one. Our practical world is not without light from the beyond. We do not have complete confidence in the world. The dangers, denials and doubts which surround the little island of life like a sea, challenge us to seek across the unknown. Ideals of love, truth and freedom lure us on to the shores of the beyond.

A real life is one which strives to be honest, to be in touch with the truths of our Self and the world. It is a life of growth, transformation of outlook, improvement of understanding. A sensible and creative life moves ever closer to the basic realities of existence and the universal concerns of history. When man finally stands on his unfailing inner strength, the rock of Self, then all doubts vanish, all bonds are broken, and he attains that imperturbable serenity of mind, that confidence of character, which is the true fruit of wisdom.

The question is often raised as to how and why avidya or ignorance arose? How did consciousness, which is pure and universal, come to be clouded and fragmented? Yoga does not claim to explain the mystery of existence. Ignorance has no beginning in time. Time exists only in the mind. Consciousness is logically prior to time and change. Time is born with our experience of change. The question is within maya and truly illogical.

Though avidya has no beginning in time and there is no explanation for the manifestation of plurality and change out of the Silent Deep, yet it is a matter of fact that false knowledge or ignorance does come to an end. There is no logical explanation for the world. The best that has been said in this connection is that the world is a play or sport of the spirit; it is the manifestation of the delight of existence. In our life, too, we want to play, to do things, and not to work, i.e. to be ourselves, to express our "feelings". We say this is our real life, but real life is the life of the spirit. This concept may not be comprehensible and may even sound cruel until we rise to the plane of truth and see things in a different perspective.

SPIRIT, PURUSHA AND NATURE, PRAKRITI

In yoga, pure consciousness is often called *Purusha*, or the person. *Purusha* literally means the indwelling spirit of man. It is also termed intelligence *(chit)*, or knowledge *(jnana)*. It is the pure subject, the seer or the *drashta*.

Nature, or *prakriti*, is opposed to consciousness or Purusha. Nature is process or phenomena; it is both matter and mind. *Prakriti* means the original principle of change. It is also called *Maya*, the creative energy of the universe. It is the object, the seen or the *drishya*. Prakriti is also called *Pradhana*, or the original source of nature.

Patanjali maintains a plurality of Purushas and a dualism between consciousness and nature, which are rejected by the integral yogic tradition of the Gita and the Upanishads. According to them, nature is the dynamic aspect, the creative power of the spirit which is one. The universe is seen as a play of power, an emanation from the silent transcendent Spirit. Reality is one; it is manifested on different levels as matter, life, mind, intellect and consciousness. The pure spirit is infinite and remains infinite after all manifestation.

Nature, or the creative power of spirit, evolves through several steps into this manifold universe. The yogic concept of nature and its evolution have been widely misunderstood. To avoid misunderstanding, we have to give up the commonsense notions of matter, mind and evolution.

Patanjali succinctly gives a profound definition of nature. He defines nature as constituted of the three principles of *sattva, rajas* and *tamas* (intelligibility or perceptibility, activity and resistance) and as that which evolves into the sensibles and sense organs for the experience and freedom of man.

The three basic constituents of nature (sattva, rajas and tamas) are called the *gunas* or principles. The gunas are usually translated as qualities, but are better understood as the strands which together make up the fabric of nature.

Nature exists in two states, potential and manifest. As a potential, indiscrete, undifferentiated entity it is called *avyakta*. As manifested, differentiated and manifold, it is called *vyakta*. In the unmanifested state the three gunas are in equilibrium. Manifestation takes place due to an imbalance of these factors.

The concept of the gunas is difficult but must be grasped if ‹one is to have a proper understanding of yoga.

THE GUNAS

If we analyze nature as an unknown entity, we discover three basic factors. We come to know things as a result of some kind of activity. Activity means transfer of energy, a state of change. All perceptions, whether external or internal, are due to activity. This activity, energy or dynamic principle in nature is the *rajas* of yoga. It can also be called the mutative principle. There is a potential or conserved state before and after all activity. For instance, in acquiring knowledge, the last activity occurs in the brain where what is known then resides in a potential state. This is the *tamas* or the conservative principle. We know objects when the potential energy or the static principle called the brain undergoes change or transference of energy. When the conservative principle is stimulated into activity we have·the sentient state. This is the *sattva* of yoga. It may be called the sentient principle, or the principle of awareness.

The three principles of sattva, rajas, and tamas are found in all phenomena of nature, mental or physical, in differing proportions. They are the basic stuff of nature. In other words nature is conceived and felt basically as energy, resistance and intelligibility.

These three factors always coexist in different degrees. There is no energy, whether it be in waves or quanta, without resistance. There is no activity, without some kind of awareness or 'prehension' however faint that may be. There is no absolute stillness, staticity or mass.

When these three factors are held in perfect equilibrium, there is no manifestation or knowledge of things. At that time the knower is self-aware or established in his own Self. This is the Person, Pure Self, or metempiric Consciousness of yoga.

Things or phenomena are constituted of the three principles of intelligibility, activity and resistance. Things are known or can be known, i.e. they have being, or intelligibility. They are also mixtures of energy and resistance, i.e. partly congealed energy. Science deals with rajas and tamas, energy and mass, but takes no cognizance of sattva, or the sentient principle.

Phenomena differ because of the different proportions in which the gunas enter into their composition. Where tamas is dominant things are more solid and massive, where rajas is dominant there is more activity and vitality, where sattva is dominant there is more manifestation or revelation, as in mental operations. In what we call matter, life is latent and mind sub-latent; in life mind is latent and superconsciousness sub-latent; in mind or selfconsciousness super-consciousness is latent.

Pure Consciousness or Purusha is beyond the gunas, i.e. transcendent; it is singular and not plural. It is reflected in the mind which therefore appears conscious, like a mirror reflecting the sun.

EVOLUTION

Nature evolves from the unmanifest state, or avyakta, to the manifest state, or vyakta, in several stages. The order of evolution is logical and not chronological. Evolution takes place in two spheres, the subjective, i.e. the empirically subjective, and the objective. On the subjective side, the first evolute is the pure "I" feeling (asmita or buddhi); from it evolves the dynamic 'I' feeling or ego. This is the

'I' feeling or self-awareness which is always related to some condition or other of the body and mind. From the ego comes the mind which is a faculty with a variety of functions including the subconscious workings of the body. Life force is a subconscious activity of the mind. The different sense organs, rather sense faculties (*indriyas*), the five of action and the five of perception, also evolve from the mind. They are diversifications of the powers of knowing and acting which are found in all sentient beings in either rudimentary or developed form.

On the objective side, the first evolute of nature is the cosmic "I" feeling, Ego, (*mahat*); this evolves into the five infrasensibles (*tanmatras*); they evolve into the five sensibles (*bhutas*) or 'elements'. The gross world is a combination of the five sensibles (*mahabhuta*).

The *tanmatras* are the superfine movements of energy behind the perception of the five sensible qualities (touch, taste, smell, sound and light) which correspond to the five senses. Yoga calls these the sensibles, elements and they are technically known as earth, water, fire, air and ether. These are not to be confounded with what their names usually imply. The gross sensibles or objects of sense are a mixture of these five sensibles in different proportions.

I have given what I consider to be the most authentic view of the order and categories of evolution. There are variations in other schools; sometimes the differences are due to different methods of analysis, sometimes to lack of understanding.

The order of evolution and the evolutes can now be given in a graphic form as below:

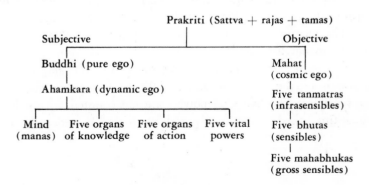

The evolutes of the different orders and prakriti are called tattvas or principles. Tattva literally means 'thatness', i.e. the real. Tattvas are the basic classes of things, or categories of existence. The orders correspond to the levels of perception during concentration. The tattvas are not abstract concepts but perceptions.

The world is one. The real is one but it is a tapering sort of reality; it tapers, level by level, from the gross sensibles or objects below to the finer and superfine realms above. In the Gita and the Upanishads the world is compared to a tree with the roots above in the heavens and the spreading branches and leaves below.

The tattvas are related to one another as creating and created. According to this principle of relationship, nature is divided into three categories, namely: 1) Nature that is uncreated and creates; 2) Nature that is created and creates, 3) Nature that is created and does not create. Nature that creates and is uncreated is called prakriti. Nature that creates and is created is called *prakriti-vikriti*. Nature that is created and does not create is called vikriti.

Avyakta is prakriti; all the other tattvas from the ego to the mind on the subjective side and from the ego to the tanmatras on the objective side are prakriti-vikritis; while ·the sense organs, the vital powers and the sensibles are all vikriti. Purusha is also a tattva, a principle. But it neither creates nor is created.

Creation in the sense given above means transformation or development. The fourfold division of principles according to creativity reminds one of the exactly similar division made by the medieval Irish philosopher John Scotus (9th century), who was influenced by Greek thought. It is interesting to speculate on the similarity of the fourfold divisions of nature according to yoga and Scotus.

The tattvas, it will be seen, are 24 in number, namely, 1) prakriti, 2) mahat and buddhi (they are the same principle, the "I" feeling, cosmic and individual), 3) ahamkara (the empirical self), 4) mind, 14) the ten sense organs, 19) the five tanmatras, 24) the five sensibles. The five vital powers are not counted separately; they are distinguished functionally and are included under the unconscious activities of the mind. The five gross sensibles or what we usually call material objects are not new principles or tattvas, being combinations in different degrees of the five sensibles.

The tattvas are emanations from prakriti, the original principle. They are like the emanations of Plotinus. Tattvas are discovered by meditation. As concentration deepens, the world of many forms and qualities is perceived in their finer or subtle aspects as forms of energy and finally as the activity of the Cosmic Mind. On the subjective side, the sense faculties become withdrawn and absorbed into the mind, the mind into the dynamic self, the dynamic self into the pure "I" feeling, and the "I" feeling into the unmanifest. Beyond the unmanifest is the pure consciousness, the metempiric consciousness. This is purusha which is often counted as the 25th tattva or principle. The stages of involution correspond to levels of meditation.

I want to repeat again that before trying to understand the yoga concept of nature and evolution, we should relinquish our commonsense views of matter and mind. Modern physical theories provide a better basis of approach.

Finally, nature, i.e. the process, is not without purpose. Its goal is to lead men through experience to spiritual freedom. In nature we see the progressive manifestation of intelligence and the gradual emancipation of consciousness. This is the universal goal of history.

Man is born in chains but struggles through history toward the freedom beyond.

Yoga gives a teleological explanation of change and a philosophical view of history. Nature is not a blind movement; a deep and secret purpose draws it forward to divine fulfillment in man.

I would like to reemphasize here for the sake of clarity the salient points of the yoga view of nature and evolution.

Nature or prakriti is an original principle and not created. The school of Patanjali regards it as an independent principle distinct from purusha or consciousness, but the integral and broad yoga maintains that nature is a power of consciousness, its dynamic and creative aspect, which manifests the visible universe through stages of development. The stages are not chronological but logical and can be always known through a trained mind.

The visible universe, despite its limitless scope and bewildering variety, communicates itself to us in the language of the five senses. The active principles behind the five distinct groups of sensations are forms of radiant energy and are called earth, water, fire, air and space, which are technical names, not to be confused with what they stand for in common parlance. Our ordinary perceptions are composite, i.e. they are mixtures of the five different factors or elements in varying proportions. The yogi can isolate and recognize the separate causal factors through higher concentration.

The ordinary objects are only incessant series of mutations and appear to have enduring forms and stability due to the inability of the untrained mind to notice changes of extreme rapidity and subtlety. The world is a perpetual emanation from a source of radiant energy and can be so perceived through developed concentration.

Our knowledge of the world is a knowledge of motion. But motion as noted above co-exists with the principles of resistance and perceptibility. All motion is rhythmic and intermittent and has a degree of perceptibility. Activity, resistance and intelligibility are the three strands or gunas (sattva, rajas, tamas) which make up the fabric of nature.

The different stages of nature's development are relative to the powers of perception. Yoga is thoroughly empirical though the range of experience on which it bases its formulations is infinitely wider than the world of common percipients. The tattvas are realities on different levels of perception.

Space and time are not objective realities but constructs of understanding. The extremely rapid changes are spread out in several dimensions due to the incapacity of the mind to comprehend them as they are. That which is open to common view is present, the rest is past and future. Language is full of abstract and empty concepts like time and space; they are practically valid but have no objective existence.

Finally the activity which gives rise to the world of experience is, at bottom, mental in character, i.e. mind is logically prior to material appearance. The universe is the development of the cosmic mind.

Natural evolution in time is purposive, being the progressive manifestation of Intelligence. Emancipation of consciousness from the bondage of matter is the goal of nature and destiny of man. On higher levels of life, evolution proceeds through the appeal that love and beauty, truth and freedom, strength and dignity make to the human heart. Nature rejects through the choice of man, her instrument, ugliness in all form, in body, mind and spirit. Man grows through imitation of the great. The movement is slow and often painful but inevitable. Nature holds secretly, in the depths of her heart, a profound concern for spiritual values. Truth and beauty, love and strength, harmony and peace will progressively triumph over falsehood and ugliness, hate and weakness, discord and conflict. Creativity is the actualization of a divine idea and takes place through the natural selection of higher values.

Theories of nature and evolution which a few scientists like J. Huxley and Teilhard du Chardin are framing today are faint and unclear echoes of the yoga view.

MAN, HIS BONDAGE AND FREEDOM

Man is born in chains but struggles toward freedom. His chains are his illusions which rest on the basic metaphysical ignorance called avidya, which is confusion of Self with non-self, spirit with nature. Freedom lies in Self-knowledge. Freedom is not of the soul, but freedom is the very nature of Self.

Ignorance makes man forget his true identity and confuse it with the changing processes of body and mind. Such identification constitutes his apparent nature. The Mundaka Upanishad describes the twofold nature of man, his bondage and his freedom in the following manner:

Two birds of beautiful plumage, close companions to each other, dwell on the self-same tree. Of them, one eats the sweet fruits; the other without eating watches silently.

Attached to the same tree and held in bondage, the individual sorrows for lack of freedom; but when he sees the other, the worshipped, transcendent Divine Being and His greatness, his sorrow passes away.

When the seer perceives the golden colored Divine Person, the Lord and Creator of the Universe then he, the knower, shakes off sin and virtue and, pure of all stain, attains the supreme identity.

He who is the Life of life manifests Himself in all beings. Knowing him well the wise man draws back from creeds and words. Such an one takes delight in Self, dwells in Self and is active; he is the best among the Knowers of Brahman.

The above verses give the profound truth of man's dual nature, real and apparent, his bondage and freedom.

The silent bird that witnesses without eating is man's real nature; the other bird, its companion, is a reflection of the silent Spirit. The tree is the body-mind complex. As long as man remains ignorant of his transcendent nature, he has no freedom and cannot be happy. When he discovers his true nature, he not only goes beyond all sorrow but finds positive delight in Self. He sees the same Self in all, the unity behind all plural appearances, and he is active in the world.

The separateness of things or their manifoldness is formal, i.e. it is an appearance on every level of existence, material, vital, mental and spiritual. Plurality of things is skin-deep.

The various forms we see in the world look distinct to our eyes but science reveals that they are configurations of the same universal stuff or field of energy. The distinctions and the boundaries of things as we know them in everyday life are due to the limitation of our senses and exist in a certain focus and scale of perception.

The same life, starting from some primitive manifestation, has assumed innumerable forms.

Mind also is universal. Apart from the higher yogic perceptions, the many kinds of parapsychological phenomena which have engaged the attention of critical investigators for a long time point clearly to the unity of mind, the individual mind being a single portion of it.

A few years ago in a symposium on parapsychology held by the Third Programme of the BBC, a number of psychologists spoke on several aspects of this subject. The last speaker in the series endeavored to organize and sum up the facts presented by formulating a few theories. He said that the phenomena considered led to the conclusion that mind is like an ocean, one and universal, and that the individual mind is a part of it like a wave upon a vast expanse of water.

Parapsychological investigations, as well as scientific considerations, lead to revision of the commonsense notions of time and causality, but this subject is beyond the scope of the present discussion.

Further it is not possible to maintain any radical distinction between the various levels of existence. Matter, both physical and chemical, merges into life; biological forces merge into the unconscious mind; the unconscious merges into the conscious functions. Existence is continuous on different levels and from one level to another. It is one nature dividing itself into many forms and classes.

Finally we discover the perfect and basic unity in spirit and consciousness. The Upanishads declare that there are not many things in the world; the Reality is one and is, at core, Spirit. The distinctions are merely transformations of one original principle. They are matters of language and form (nama rupa) rather than of substance. Distinctions are linguistic and formal.

Freedom lies in the clear integral perception of the underlying unity of the universe.

KARMA AND REBIRTH

Karma is one of the basic principles of yoga and oriental philosophy. It is a doctrine regarding human bondage and freedom. The word has become a commonplace in many languages, but its popular meaning is a ridiculous caricature of its true sense and intention.

Yoga is pragmatic. Beliefs are true in so far as they can be verified in experience. No theory can be completely validated in the strictest sense, dissolving all doubts or the possibilities of doubt. But a belief is tenable and worthy of credence as long as it stands the test of experience and explains facts which remain otherwise inexplicable. The validity of a concept or belief rests on its practical consequences (arthakriyakaritva).

Karma is no blind belief. It is both a fact and a theory to interpret the life and experience of an individual. It does not make everything clear. What theory of life ever does? But it makes far more sense to our reason, pure and practical, than does any other hypothesis. In essence, the doctrine expresses the fact of human bondage and determinism yet asserts at the same time man's ability to achieve freedom by his own effort. This is the substance of karma, which is a fact of experience.

Karma affirms the continuity and progress of life and gives the kind of answer which is adequate to the demands of our moral sense, which is otherwise perplexed by the enigma of life and the chance and caprice of its fortunes.

The word karma literally means "action" in the broadest sense. It has many other meanings. In its strictly technical and limited sense it means the action of a sentient individual as well as the result or effect of such an action upon the individual. The result may be in the shape of a habit or tendency or disposition left by an action or in the form of a reaction caused by it. The habit or tendency created by an action may remain dormant or invisible for a long or short time in the depths of one's mind. This is known as karmasamskara or samskara. The dormant karmasamskara is known as the preconscious and unconscious in depth psychology.

The doctrine of *karma* offers a philosophical explanation of the life and experience of an individual in terms of a moral law operative in the universe and not as the working out of a blind chance or fate, or the fiat of a whimsical Ruler of the world. The individual is the maker of his own destiny; he determines by his own action his future life and experience, his happiness and misery, his success and failure. This dictum needs to be seen and examined in its proper context in order to avoid common misunderstandings.

We feel, all of us, that we are more or less free, within limits, to shape our lives and determine our careers by our own efforts. At the same time, we are also aware that we are limited, determined and fashioned by situations and circumstances beyond our control. Further there are within us hidden depths and sunken habits of thought, feeling and desire which govern our will and action.

We must not forget the universal context of our individualistic existence in our attempts to understand the meaning of karma.

We, as individuals, are patterns of processes in a universal flow of energy just as any other forms are. And though as individuals we have a history of our own, a career which has some sort of self-direction and self-determination from within, yet being part of a cosmic tide, we are subject to its influence.

Further, karma belongs to the world of maya, that is, what we call our practical world. In discussing it we must not confuse the two levels of truth and experience, the transcendental and the phenomenal.

The sense of freedom and individuality which we have may not be philosophically tenable or understood, but they are the presuppositions of our conduct. Karma works within such presuppositions.

Viewed from the transcendental or the highest standpoint of yogic experience, the will of an individual is never free. Freedom belongs to the universal Self alone. The Self is freedom. The individual will is always determined. Philosophers have debated the question of human freedom and determination endlessly without coming to any solution. The problem is insoluble since it is wrongly posed.

Philosophically speaking there can be only one will or force which is free, namely, the will or force which is universal and identical with the world. In the measure that the will of an individual is in harmony with the universal will and in the degree that an individual is aware of his identification with the Cosmic Self, to that measure and degree can he be regarded as free.

However, the discussion of karma is meaningful in the empirical context; but this context is much more extensive than we suppose. The doctrine of karma is not limited to our present life alone. It extends on the one hand to a beginingless past and on the other to an indeterminate future. Further, it includes all those experiences which are supernormal.

The doctrine of rebirth is part of the principle of karma. It is necessary at this stage to remove some confusion in connection with rebirth or reincarnation; confusion which pretends to be some kind of a logical argument against it but which rests essentially on a misunderstanding. It is claimed that since there is no substantive entity called the soul, the ego being an illusory notion, there cannot be any transmigration or rebirth. Neither yoga nor Buddhism assert that there is an individual soul substance, yet they maintain the doctrine of karma and rebirth.

The confusion arises from an uncritical materialism and a naive misunderstanding. Though there may be no substantive things or persons in the world yet we talk as if there are, because we see continuity in patterns of processes. There is no substantive individual even now, not to speak of one going from here to the hereafter. Yet just as a physical process as an individual pattern exists and endures for a length of time, so also a psychical process may continue independently apart from its association with a gross physical form and for a longer time.

That mind or psyche can exist apart from the body, and that it can know and act without the sense media, are not matters of speculation or wishful thinking but facts of experience which cannot be denied except by those who choose to close their eyes. Mind or a mental process can exist independently of the body and can also be associated with a series of bodies.

Mind and matter are two levels of the same principle, they are not two absolutely distinct entities. But mind is more fundamental than matter. This is the conclusion not only of many philosophers who rely on reasoning but also of many scientists who have been led to it by the discoveries of modern science. Old fashioned matter or body has become an abstract idea of the mind. What exists objectively is energy. But energy is an unknown entity, the existence of which is recognized only during its state of change and as it is manifested in different forms, such as light, heat, magnetism, electricity, etc. The only activity, work or energy that we know directly is the activity of our mind. On purely philosophical grounds, the basic energy or stuff of the universe is best conceived in psychological terms.

Plato said, "The ether is the mother and reservoir of visible creation — an invisible and formless eidos, the most difficult of comprehension and partaking somehow of the nature of mind." (Timaeus)

Several modern scientists and biologists view the primary stuff of the world as having properties of life and mind.

The doctrine of rebirth is not confined to yoga and Buddhism alone. It was widely current in the ancient world among the Egyptians, the Greeks, the Jews, the Neo-Platonists, the early Christians, the Arabs and others. As a philosophical theory it has appealed to many thinkers and scientists who are critical of all beliefs. The skeptical philosopher Hume remarked: "Metempsychosis is the only anti-materialistic system which philosophy could hearken to." Thomas Huxley, the great biologist, said: "There is nothing in the anology of nature against it and very much to support it."

Not only is there no logical argument against rebirth but philosophically it is the only rational explanation of our life and the most cogent answer to our moral questions that we can think of.

Karma views the present life not as an isolated incident but as an episode in the larger career of our soul. Though our individual life has no beginning in time yet we can trace back from it our past existences which have made us what we are today. It is possible according to yoga, to recover the memory of our past life through meditation. If we can free ourselves from the preoccupations which tie our attention to the interests of the present life and body, our mind ranges over a wide area and recollects impressions and experiences long forgotten and hidden in its subconscious depths. The childhood experiences of our present life are not far removed in years yet how many years of analysis does it take to recover some of them!

The life we live now is one link in a long chain; it is the result of our thoughts and actions in the previous existence. Though our present life is determined by the past, it is not an absolute determination, for we can alter its course within limits. We never lose our freedom completely, and there is always the possibility that we can attain complete freedom by discovering our true identity through knowledge.

Recounting an ancient view, Patanjali asserts that our actions in the past life determine three things in particular. They are first, the kind of species in which we are born; second, the duration of our present life; and third, the nature of our experiences.

In our attempt to find reasons for the general course of our life, our health and happiness, our talents and character, our success and failure, we generally fall back upon explanations of three or four kinds. We attribute it either to heredity, to environmental factors, to the will of God or to chance. Of course, we do not altogether deny our own responsibility.

Of these, chance is no explanation really but a confession of ignorance. The theory of God's will is rationally untenable and morally repugnant. Hereditary and environmental factors as well as the fact of our own choice throw some light but leave most things in the dark. Some facts even conflict with these theories. Above all they do not rescue life from the sense of absurdity and injustice which weigh upon it in general. To many, life is a cruel joke. We look for an explanation that is more comprehensive and a light that is redeeming.

The hereditary explanation of life within a materialistic framework does not conflict with karma for according to it, we are drawn as it were by a kind of psychic gravitation to the environments and situations where our deep-seated wishes and inclinations might find or have hopes of finding their best expression and fulfillment.

Karma is an expression of moral law. What we sow, we reap—not only in this life, but also in others. Honesty is the best policy. We cannot be happy by making others unhappy. We have to pay a price for everything we get. Persons who have success by wrong means have tension along with their comforts and pleasures, which are more matters of sensation than anything else. One becomes less of a man through deceit and selfishness. The more we become estranged by our actions from the truth of the Self, the more unhappiness, anxiety and fear we create for ourselves.

There is no simple one-to-one correspondence between our action and its result as is popularly supposed. But by a wrong act we suffer contraction of our personality and freedom, thus lessening our capacity for peace and happiness. I want to quote once more the profound sanskrit saying which has the wisdom of long experience:

"By injustice men prosper, gain what they desire, and triumph over their enemies, but finally they are destroyed at their very roots."

No great achievement is accomplished through cleverness. Love brings love, hatred hatred. This is the moral law; its operation is subtle but is as true as that of physical law. We cannot be healthy by violating the laws of health, nor can we be happy and free by breaking the law of our growth. This is the heart of the law of karma. Its application is not easy to see. The more perceptive and clearsighted we become through rational and ethical self-discipline, by following the truth of our being, the more distinctly we realize the inviolability of its operation

Many today would have fared better if they thought more of integrity than of integration.

Apropos the subject of life's determination, I want to present a few facts which substantiate Patanjali's view. It is likely that some of my readers have some acquaintance with astrology. It is not an exact science, nor is it right to pay it undue attention but now and then astonishing instances of character-reading and foreknowledge of events are found on the basis of horoscopes. Jung used to consult horoscopes at times to understand the nature of his patients. Some of his followers still do.

I have witnessed a number of cases where competent astrologers in India, without knowing anything about the persons concerned except the hour, date and place of their birth have made accurate predictions of their marriages, children, siblings, travels, achievements, riches and career and finally the date and manner of their death. These predictions cannot be explained unless things are determined in some fashion hidden from common observation.

But karma is not fatalistic. It calls on men to see clearly the facts of their determination and with that in view to depend on their own efforts without sinking into a hopeless acceptance of life's misfortunes. There is a future for all.

Our present life is not absolutely determined. It has been compared to a game of bridge. The cards have been dealt out; we cannot change them. But how we play our hand depends on us. We can play well or poorly; we can make the best use of our opportunities or miss them.

Karma maintains that we are all evolving through many births and numerous experiences into the freedom of the Self. Every man has the power of the spirit behind him; through faith and action he can manifest the power and break the bondage of the past.

The meaning and necessity of many things in our present life cannot be understood unless we view it as a chapter in the long book of our experience. Modern psychology is leading toward that kind of understanding. Self-analysis and free association, without any pre-conceived theories of mind or categories of explanation, will reveal many mysteries of the psyche and reasons for much of the suffering and tension of modern man will be found in the operation of laws more profound than are generally recognized.

ACTION AND FREEDOM

In studying yoga one often comes across the expression "the bondage of karma." As we have already noted, the original meaning of karma is action. From this many jump to the conclusion that yoga is renunciation of action and pursuit of contemplation alone.

But the aim of yoga is not to relinquish action. Action is not opposed to freedom. Freedom is knowledge or wisdom and is opposed to ignorance alone. Bondage of karma is the bondage of ignorance and of the blind, mechanical, self-centered action which comes from it. Nobody can give up action entirely, nor is it necessary or right to do so. The higher life of contemplation is made possible through action. The highest life is not without action; it is a life where action is combined with wisdom.

The aim of yoga is to attain freedom of Being through decon-ditioning. Any thought or action which deconditions us, removes our illusions about our nature and Self and brings us into closer touch with reality is yogic action and therefore spiritual. Action which strengthens illusion or ignorance and limits freedom is unspiritual. A good meal which releases us from hunger and helps us attain the higher ends of life is a spiritual act. It is not activity that binds but the wrong attitude toward action. The wise man finds the silence and calmness of eternity in the din and whirl of action. He sees inaction in action.

This is the gist of the karma yoga as told in the Gita.

III
PRACTICE

III

PRACTICE

HATHA YOGA

IN THE PREVIOUS SECTION I have mentioned hatha yoga in general terms in the context of the broad and integral culture of yoga. Here I am presenting a specific and detailed account of its history, aims, principles and practices, adequate and clear enough for understanding and practice by the general public.

Interest in hatha yoga is widespread in the West today and is daily growing; articles and books on the subject are pouring into the market while libraries in the largest cities can hardly keep up with the demand. Despite all this, clear and intelligent ideas on the subject are hard to find.

Hatha yoga is a system of health and hygiene involving both body and mind. It aims at the whole man for his full development and self-realization. It takes into account not only the proper growth, strength and tone of the different muscles of the body but also the efficiency and function of the basic factors of constitutional health, namely, the inner organs and the glands. Finally it emphasizes emotional balance and a mature outlook on life, for in the long run the health which is not mental health is no health at all.

The hatha yoga exercises were first developed as a preparation for the yoga of contemplation; yet in later times elaborate techniques

99

and methods of health and hygiene were evolved which could be followed for their own sake, apart from any high spiritual motive. The purely physical aspect of this yoga thus came to be known as the *Ghatastha* yoga, or the yoga of the physical body.

The original meaning of hatha yoga is the yoga of force or physical violence, i.e., the physical and vital control of the body by physiological means for purposes of higher concentration. Later on, the word hatha came also to symbolize the two biomotor processes of the body, the energy-consuming and the energy-acquiring, which are called respectively the sun *(ha)* and the moon *(tha)* principles. According to this explanation, hatha yoga aims to balance and harmonize these two forces by means of breath control, which again is accessory to higher contemplation.

From the earliest times the yogis emphasized balance — balance between body, mind and spirit. An allround development of personality is not possible without constitutional health. An ancient yoga text declares: *The Self of man cannot be attained by the weak; the aspirant after yoga must be disciplined, strong, firm and intelligent.*

One of India's great sons, poet, philosopher, humanist and Nobel-Prize winner Rabindranath Tagore, who belonged to the integral spiritual tradition of India, once remarked that a complete man should be vitally savage and mentally civilized. A fully developed and complete individual should have the keenness of perception and the thrill of a child in its contact with nature; at the same time his mind should be goverened by civilized values.

Proper attention to body is a spiritual act. It helps to free the mind from physical bondage. Many so-called spiritual teachers who look askance at hatha yoga but who are often preoccupied with their bodies, relying so easily and quickly on drugs and surgery, are thoughtless. They would be better physically and spiritually if they had practiced a little bit of hatha yoga.

A brilliant intellect in a sick body devoid of the capacity for strong feeling and sensation, and a superbly developed physique with a dull mind and without subtle perceptions are, neither of them, ideal or desirable conditions.

Hatha yoga is based on a body of empircal knowledge built up in the course of centuries. Long, continued observation and experiment enabled the yogis to build up a system of health and hygiene eminently fitted not only to keep the body healthy, supple and strong but also to prolong youthfulness, delay aging and decay, and to make the body resistant to disease.

HATHA YOGA IN MODERN INDIA AND THE WEST

Hatha yoga has continued to be practiced in India by several groups who have passed their knowledge from teacher to pupil without disruption for over tens of centuries. A few dedicate themselves exclusively to mastering and improving its techniques, while many others, whose work and interests do not permit such exclusive concentration, follow it along with other pursuits, thus invigorating and enriching their life far beyond ordinary measure.

The various techniques and theories of hatha yoga have evolved through the practice and experience of a large body of teachers over many hundred years, during which time the effects of these exercises upon different kinds of individuals has been under continuous observation. This serves to assure us that hatha yoga is, in every respect, a superior method of physical hygiene and culture, more reliable than modern systems which have not gone through the test of time and which are partial and external in their outlook and application.

Hatha yoga techniques and theories came to be formulated, organized and presented in a number of texts. Not many of the ancient texts are available today. Of those which are in existence, many are still in manuscript form, held by the libraries of different institutions. Only a few have been printed and published, of which the best known are the HATHA DIPIKA, SIVA SAMHITA, GORAKSHA SAMHITA and GHERANDA SAMHITA. All have been translated into English. None of these books are very old, the earliest only dating back to the thirteenth century. These books are short, cryptic and often full of hyperbolic claims. They cannot be properly appraised, understood and followed without expert guidance.

It is also to be noted that the creative and empirical spirit of India gradually disappeared in later times for a variety of reasons, so that many vital truths and ideas came to be mixed with fairy tales and fantasies. Hard, rigid attitudes took the place of the old flexible and open minded inquiry.

The scientific and creative exposition of hatha yoga in our time is due mostly to the work of two distinguished yogis, Yogi Madhavdas and Shyam Sundar Goswami. Both came from old cultured families in the same district of Bengal.

Madhavdas dedicated himself to yoga early in life, travelled on foot all through India eleven times over a period of thirty years in search of yogic knowledge, and spent nearly 20 years practicing yoga in the remote Himalayas. Finally, after almost sixty years of itinerant life, Madhavdas settled down in an ashrama on the banks of the river Narmada, near Guzrat in western India. This was toward the close of the last century; he was then over eighty years old.

A group of disciples gathered round him in the ashrama for instruction, among whom was one who later translated Tagore's Nobel Prize-winning book of poems GITANJAL or SONG OFFERINGS from the original Bengali into Guzrati with Madhavdas' help. Two other students, Swami Kuvalayanand (then a medical doctor under the name of J. G. Gune) and Shri Yogendra founded, after Madhavdas' death, two institutes in Bombay to impart instruction in hatha yoga and to conduct research under modern methods of observation and experiment. Books and journals have been published from the institutes and their work has helped to spread the knowledge and practice of yoga in India and abroad.

Shyam Sundar Goswami was the disciple of a yogi of extraordinary powers named Balaki Bharati. As a boy, Shyam Sundar Goswami was weak and prone to illness. In his search for health and strength he began experimenting with various eastern and western systems of physical culture. None proved quite satisfactory, especially with regard to building resistance to disease. Finally he came upon hatha yoga, and under the instruction of Balaki Bharati, he improved his health, strength, body control and resistance to disease phenomenally. Later he established a center for yoga culture in Calcutta where he trained a number of students in advanced yogic exercises of external and internal control. Goswami travelled to different parts of India and later made lecture and demonstration tours of Europe, the United States, Japan and many other countries. In 1949, he and one of his most advanced students attended the World Congress for Physical Culture at Lingiad, Sweden, where they lectured on the yoga methods and gave demonstrations. Soon after, at the request of a deputation of physicians and other persons who had become enthusiastic, a school was established in Stockholm, giving theoretical and practical instruction in yoga.

Shyam Sundar Goswami, who is deeply versed in both western and eastern methods of physical education, has written a book on hatha yoga entitled HATHA YOGA, AN ADVANCED METHOD OF PHYSICAL EDUCATION AND CONCENTRATION. This work is modern, cogent and the most comprehensive, definitive treatment of hatha yoga to be found in the western world today. It is also the most completely illustrated book.

Yoga in various forms spread early to many Asian countries and parts of Europe. Today it has found its way to the farthest corners of the western world, including North and South America. Its adherents include princes, aristocrats, generals, businessmen, doctors, lawyers, artists, dancers, writers and politicians. England, with its long, close association with India, has been one of the principal channels through which yoga has come to the modern West. Many British officers during their stay in India became impressed by yoga and were among the first to introduce it in a practical form to the West. Mr. Yeats Brown, a British army officer, long resident in India and author of THE LIVES OF A BENGAL LANCER, was drawn to yoga and wrote a popular book on the subject.

Recently another retired British intelligence officer, Sir Paul

Dukes, who learned yoga from an oriental in pre-revolutionary Russia, wrote a book on hatha yoga in which he discusses yoga's influence on Russia in the last century and its effect upon many Russian philosophers and mystical teachers, among whom he mentions Merishkowsky, Berdyaev, Gurdjieff and Ouspensky.

Yoga appeared in the U.S.A. more than fifty years ago. In 1909, in a lecture delivered before the Philosophical Association at Columbia University entitled "The Energies of Men," Prof. William James mentioned that a friend of his, who had been given to chronic depression, fatigue and ill health, had attained remarkable results from the practice of yoga. After six months of regular and devoted practice, he was a changed man who had plenty of surplus energy and needed much less rest, sleep and food than formerly. The article was later published in a book called THE ENERGIES OF MEN AND THE GOSPEL OF RELAXATION. The book, however, omits many details of the original lecture which can be found in its entirety in The Philosophical Review.

Tributes to yoga appear in books, magazines and newspapers almost every day. In a recent publication Father Dechanet, a French Benedictine monk who was abbot of a monastery in the former Belgian Congo, records how yoga, with its relaxing and calming effect on the mind, helped him not only to attain a new feeling of physical well-being but also aided him in his prayers and meditations. Though the Father has some misconceptions about spiritual yoga, his account is rare in that it is both sensible and civilized. Most books on the market are crude in their approach, containing accounts and sweeping generalizations that are both dogmatic and distorted.

Hatha yoga is a rational and comprehensive system of health and self culture. It is not the clownish acrobatics or vulgar performance to which some tend to reduce it. Practice of the various techniques of yoga no doubt gives one extraordinary powers over the body, but character, serenity of mind and even health in the long run cannot be attained by mere physical postures. Those who so preach, mislead others.

Diverse types of physical exercise were developed in ancient India. The Encyclopaedia of Indian Physical Culture, published in 1955, records and illustrates many of them: weight-lifting, discus and javelin throwing, exercises with bars, rings, poles and maces, wrestling and so on. But hatha yoga was not evolved to build bulky specialized muscles for aggressive purpose but to assure constitutional health, and a well-proportioned, firm and flexible body, to retain youthfulness, to delay age and decay, and above all to develop the kind of body essential to a life rich and meaningful in content.

THE TECHNIQUES AND THE GENERAL FACTORS OF HEALTH

The hatha yoga techniques are collectively known as *nadi suddhi* processes, that is, processes for purifying the nerves and vitalizing the body. Purity in yoga means calmness or balance, while impurity stands for dullness and restlessness. There are four broad divisions of these techniques which are; 1) postures (*asana* and *mudra*), 2) breath control (*pranayama*), 3) dynamic contraction exercises (*charana*), 4) cleansing, special control and locking exercises (*shatkarma, bandha* and *mudra*). Of these the asanas or postures, and the pranayamas or breath-regulations, are the most well known and widely practiced.

Before going on to posture, breathing and other techniques it will be of interest to consider the hatha yoga exercises generally in relation to the basic factors of health.

The efficiency of the abdomino-thoracic structure, the internal organs and the glands, determine our health, youthfulness, vigor and longevity. This includes the spine, the thoracic and abdominal muscles, the lungs, the heart and the endocrine glands.

Spine

A firm and flexible spine is essential for health and youthfulness. A man is as old as his spine. Age bends the spine. We are all familiar with the expression "A man of strong backbone." Doctors today realize the great importance of the spine in preserving health and assuring long life. The emphasis that chiropractors and osteopaths place on the spine is well known. If the spine loses its natural spring-like curvature, if the spinal bones are not properly aligned, or if they are burdened with calcium deposits, our health and efficiency are vastly reduced. Wrong alignment and stiffness of vertebrae impair the function of nerves which issue out of vertebral apertures and control the motor and sensory activities of the different limbs. An increasingly greater number of people are today suffering from various forms of back troubles, from weak vertebrae, slipped discs and sacroiliac difficulties, which are so often due to bad posture and lack of specialized exercise. Wrong posture also interferes with the normal activities of various internal organs and reduces their efficiency.

The spinal, abdominal and respiratory muscles function as the fundamental muscles in all mammals, including man. The earliest means of locomotion and patterns of movement are connected with the spinal musculature.

An erect spinal posture is necessary for holding the thorax in the correct position. Weakness of chest muscles makes the thorax droop to the position natural for exhalation, which hampers normal breathing. On the other hand the high upraised barrel chest often developed through "muscle-building" exercises, lifts the thorax to an inspiratory position also interfering with normal breathing. Erect trunk posture and proper development and tone of the chest and abdominal muscles are important conditions for proper breathing, healthy body function, concentration and a high emotional level.

Hatha yoga is the only system which pays special attention to spine culture. The spinal exercises make the back bone firm and flexible, hold the vertebrae in position and stimulate the sympathetic nerve chains which lie embedded in the muscles of the back along the spine. The various specialized spinal and abdominal movements of hatha yoga stimulate the fundamental nerve centers and the basic muscular movements of the body, apart from producing other effects.

Breathing

Proper breathing habits are essential for health. It is the basic function of the body on which depends the proper working of every other organ. Lungs need regular and correct exercises and education as do the other limbs of the body for their healthy and optimum functioning. The civilized man in the comfortable societies of today uses only a small part of his lung capacity. As a consequence of faulty and shallow breathing, the extreme areas of the lungs remain unexercised, becoming inelastic and atrophied like muscles which grow stiff and wither away from lack of use. As breathing becomes more shallow and rapid, the heart beats more often. There is a close relationship between the rate of breathing and the rapidity of heart beats. Faulty breathing puts a severe strain on the heart. The heart muscle rests only during the interval between beats and if we shorten the interval needlessly by faulty breathing, we deprive it of its needed rest. It is like making a horse run continuously by flogging it. It can be expected to break down quickly from sheer exhaustion.

Regular and proper movement of the diaphragm is necessary for health of the various organs inside the abdominal cavity. Nature intended those organs to be stimulated by the rhythmic movement of the diaphragm which imparts to them a kind of massage. Without such stimulation, the functioning of the organs is impaired and many troubles ensue. The proper and educated movement of the diaphragm and the abdominal muscles helps to ensure healthy periods and facilitates natural childbirth.

Proper breathing improves the form and structure of the body. A few years ago, two German doctors who had been teaching and practicing yoga for years, brought out a book called "ATEMHEILKUNST" ("THE ART OF HEALING BREATH"), in which they point out, with the evidence of charts and graphs, the importance of correct breathing.

They clearly demonstrate how breathing controls the various bodily functions, and how the proper structure of the body depends on proper breathing. Unless the lungs function well, the body, especially in the trunk and the shoulders, does not have good form.

Yoga lays special emphasis on breathing exercises for both physiological and psychological reasons. Proper functioning of the lungs is essential for physical and mental well being. One can prolong life and retard the aging process through breathing.

The lungs need to be fully stretched by special exercises to maintain their full efficiency. Untrained lungs run quickly out of breath and take an unduly long time to recover, even after modest exertion. The air passages which remain stagnant due to poor breathing provide areas where bacteria find easy lodging and grow quickly. Lack of movement and faulty circulation in the lungs cause a good many colds and respiratory troubles.

Oxygen forms by far the major constituent of the body. Faulty breathing lowers vitality by depriving the body cells of their proper oxygen needs. Some researchers maintain that lack of oxygen in the tissues is a prime factor in causing cancer. They say that the body cells which are chronically cut off from oxygen supply go back to a primitive method of metabolism which causes cancerous growth. There is no doubt that faulty breathing wears out the body in many ways.

Age reduces the efficiency of the bodily organs. Breathing capacity is progressively diminished with growing years. Being the key function of life, the loss of breathing power inevitably hastens the deterioration of other organs and cells in the body. Breathing exercises retard such processes.

Slow and rhythmic breathing acquired through yoga practice slows down the heart and prevents both the unnecessary wear and tear on the body and the strain on the nervous system which come from irregular breathing. Ordinarily a man at rest breathes 17 or 18 times a minute. One who has practised yoga breathing faithfully breathes 7 to 8 times a minute. Such slow and deep breathing is restful to the nerves and cuts down the aging process.

Breathing & Psyche

The various psychic and physiological effects of regulated breathing are coming to be recognized by doctors and psychiatrists in the West.

Breathing is a bridge between the voluntary and involuntary functionings of the body, between the conscious mind and the subconscious psyche, between body and Spirit. Our breathing reflects our state of mind; elation or depression, restlessness or repose. Through proper and regulated breathing, we can gain a large measure of control over our emotions. By controlling and regulating our breath, we can do much to relax our nerves and develop powers of concentration.

Deep, rhythmic and controlled breathing has a profound effect on the whole nervous system and the psyche. Many doctors, psychiatrists and analysts today advise their patients to do some form of breathing to relieve tension. Persons have been relieved of heart conditions through regulated deep breathing The yogis discovered long ago the psychological and spiritual benefits of educated and controlled breathing. They went deep into the subject and developed it into a great art.

Heart

Heart disease is the greatest killer in America today. The reason is both physical and mental. False values, worship of false gods, estrangement from the deeper truth of our nature, the rush and hurry of the 'rat race,' create tensions which attack the heart. Diet no doubt plays its part but its role has been overstressed. Overweight and lack of exercise also contribute to heart trouble, but emotional tensions play by far the most important part in lowering vitality and causing damage to the heart. The yogis emphasize the importance of emotional balance for health. There cannot be any true integration and balance between the different demands and sides of our personality without a central purpose of life. This is the function of philosophy—to provide us with a scale of values and a perspective. Though ultimately thinking individuals cannot be very healthy without a philosophical outlook, yet physical means are not to be neglected. Yoga breathings, postures and exercises relax tension and improve the heart.

Glands

Glands, which control metabolism, growth and body functions are, as a whole, influenced by emotions. As heart disease is the greatest killer in the United States today, arthritis is the greatest crippler. The faulty function of adrenal glands in an affluent and well-nourished society is due primarily to emotional difficulties. Constant fear, resentment and anxiety, open or suppressed, deplete the glands which then fail to supply the hormones necessary to ward off arthritic attacks. Emotional trouble wears out the body so quickly that old age with all its stiffness, aches and pains sets in early. Yogic hygiene, including mental outlook, diet, and exercises, especially certain breathings and postures, improves the functioning of the glands and restores prematurely lost powers

The different yoga postures involve the body in diversified exercises, thus keeping it well-proportioned, slim and flexible. Yoga helps to reduce excess weight and tone up the muscles, especially those left untouched by ordinary strenuous exercises.

The control exercises and cleansing practices of hatha yoga are for higher breath control and breath suspension. Of these only a few are suitable for those who are interested in physical health and hygiene. The others are for specialists and are not to be recommended to the general public.

Cleanliness, both outer and inner, is an essential condition of health. Daily washings and baths, especially for persons living in warm climates and overheated rooms, keep the body free from troubles of various kinds. Much heaviness and dullness of the body and mind come from unclean habits and food. One begins to desire stimulants in order to be wakened from a feeling of torpor and sluggishness. Lightness of body and cheerfulness of mind, which stems from cleanliness, diminishes and stops the craving for strong drinks and tobacco.

Many of the intricate cleansing techniques of hatha yoga are difficult to learn; they need have no place in modern hygiene. Some results can be more easily and effectively achieved by modern methods. Further, the elaborate and intricate cleansing methods were prescribed originally for individuals who were preparing themselves for special techniques of body and nerve control and for those who had special health problems. It is not advisable for normal persons to do them either for health or spiritual progress.

Ordinary cleansing methods are important and can be easily followed by one and all.

The basic postures and breathing exercises of hatha yoga are easy to learn and follow. No instrumental or mechanical aids are necessary. They can be done by young and old alike. No matter what your age you can always improve by practicing some aspect of yoga.

There are thousands in the West today who keep themselves fit and vigorous by doing yoga exercises. Yoga postures are being increasingly incorporated into the disciplines of western physical culturists and dance instructors for promoting health, control, flexibility and versatility of body movement.

Hatha yoga shapes the body on a slender, wiry pattern, capable of great exertion and endurance, and stresses a muscular development consistent with constitutional health and vigor. Overdeveloped and hypertrophied muscles, enlarged through wrong and strenuous methods of exercise, prey like parasites on general vitality. In failing to train the lungs and heart for the increased oxygen and fuel demands of the overdeveloped body, such exercise programs bring about premature senility and death.

Its rational, psychophysical, integral approach makes hatha yoga the most suitable form of health culture for the civilized man.

FOOD, FAST AND ASCETICISM

Intelligent consideration of food and eating habits has always been important for sound health. Today, however, such attention has become a matter of paramount concern in societies where food is plentiful in both variety and richness and where temptations are too many and too easily indulged.

In matters of food, as in other matters relating to daily living only a few general principles can be laid down, for life is too complex, varied and fluid to be guided by a few formulas.

Further, even in these days of specialized and advanced knowledge, we do not know enough to have unchallengeable opinions in regard to even the most simple things. However, certain broad and sound conclusions can be drawn from reason and experience.

In matters of food, intelligent consideration as well as the "body wisdom" that comes from healthy habits are important. Civilized man, living in artificial surroundings and depending on artificial food and stimulants, has almost lost that natural instinct for the right kind of food which both animals and children possess.

By following body wisdom, developing subtle perceptions, and also from long continued observations, the yogis formulated a number of principles about food, fasting and eating, the values of which are being recognized increasingly today.

People often wonder what they should eat. The answer for most people is of course that they should eat less. They often overeat for many reasons. Overeating deforms the body, impairs health, reduces efficiency and shortens life.

There is a prevalent notion that energy, strength and vigor can be increased and maintained by a liberal intake of rich nutrients. Such a practice, followed contrary to natural instincts, often burdens the body with morbid materials, makes the blood impure and creates unhealthy conditions.

The amount of food should be cut down after the age of 35 or so. We need food for growth, for repairing the wear and tear of body tissues and for fuel purposes. We cease to grow after the age of 30 or 35, and become less active and physically playful than we were in younger years. However, our eating habits not only persist but change for the worse. We then have more means and more inclination to eat and drink. I once saw a man of enormous proportions, captain of a small Greek boat at sea, patiently cracking and eating nearly two pounds of almonds spread out on a table one afternoon shortly after lunch, "just to kill time," as his assistant explained. The captain is not a great exception.

Overeating is one of the deadliest sins according to the Hindu scriptures. They regard it as worse than dissoluteness and as a distorted version of sexuality. The tongue likes food which the stomach cannot digest. Overeating wears out the digestive organs. Food which cannot be assimilated is eliminated as refuse and that which is absorbed in excess of the needs of the body is deposited as unnecessary, burdensome and injurious fat. The noxious materials in the blood, the by-products of digestion are increased in amount. The acids and toxins and the metabolic debris released in the blood stream and the tissue fluids are not so easily expelled from the bodies of older people as from youngsters.

Gerontology is a new branch of study concerned with the aging process. Gerontologists maintain that the waste products in the body of an individual of, say 40, take nearly four or five times longer to be eliminated than those in the body of a young man of 18. Impure, weak blood of overfed individuals is a prime reason why they so often catch cold and flu and fall victims to other diseases.

Gerontologists are now turning their attention to the habits of people who lead a long and healthy life to find out the factors responsible for their health and longevity. From long experience and insight, the yogis came to certain conclusions which have been validated by those who have lived according to these principles.

One is that the amount and type of food should be changed in later years. Food should be cut down and the number of meals reduced after middle age There should be long intervals between meals. When you are in doubt whether you should eat or not, don't.

Periodic fasting, one day in the week or in a fortnight, is very beneficial for grownups. It cleanses the body and restores vitality. Take plenty of fluids in the form of diluted fruit juice or lemon water while you fast. If you feel hungry, take a light fruit or a vegetable meal in the evening.

Fasting and food regulations are also effective in curing many troubles, but they should be undertaken only under expert advice and observation.

Many persons who suffer from a variety of troubles and diseases have been cured of them while undertaking fasts for reducing weight.

Modern nutritionists have discovered that animals who are a little underfed live longer and have more vitality than those whose intake is larger.

Food should generally be moderate. Yogis say that only half the stomach should be filled with food. Of the rest, a quarter should be for water and another for air. Unless there is enough space in the stomach, the muscles cannot work; the result is indigestion. It is good as a general rule to leave the table a little hungry, especially for those who are past middle age.

Food should be fresh and clean and as far as possible unprocessed. Domestic animals are often better nutritionists than many of us whose natural and healthy instincts have been blunted and corrupted by artificial flavoring and treatment of food. Animals avoid food which has been so processed by chemical and other means as to have been denuded of its essential nutrients and vitamins, although it has been made alluring and attractive by color and scent which serve as decoys. Older people should avoid greasy and fried things which are hard on the liver.

One should reduce meat eating and give it up altogether, if possible, as one grows in years, especially if one lives in warm or hot climates. However, in considering dietary rules and changes, doctrinaire attitudes are to be avoided and attention should be given to the various factors which demand consideration, such as background, occupation, age, interest, etc. Individuals differ in their metabolic machinery, in the production and utilization of different enzymes. They further differ in their need for and assimilation of different types of protein. Fresh fish is generally a good substitute for meat.

There is a mistaken belief that vegetarianism is a creed of yoga. Food regulations as such are no essential part of yoga or true spirituality. Vegetarianism is a matter of feeling and also of consideration for health. There are many Hindus, including brahmins and monks, who will eat fish or flesh but do not kill animals. Even Buddhist monks eat meat offered to them as alms. Many great spiritual teachers ate and eat meat. Rama, Krishna and Buddha ate meat. Meat eating does not make one unspiritual, nor does vegetarianism itself make one purer or holier than others. Vegetarians are not necessarily lacking in cruelty, violence, hatred, greed, lust, ignorance or pride. And there are persons who carry the practice to insane fanatic lengths, even forcing vegetarianism on their pet animals. However, there are good reasons behind a vegetarian diet for a large number of persons, especially those in their later years who suffer from certain difficulties. It is also beneficial for many spiritual aspirants and intellectual workers. Meat and liver, rich in nutrients though they are, produce a lot of harmful toxins and poison-forming bacteria, which are not easily expelled from the body. Their reduction and elimination from the food intake make for better health.

The false notion that men need animal protein in one form or another in order to live is sometimes propagated even by doctors and nutritionists. This is not true at all. Man's earliest food consisted of plants, roots and fruits; later fish, flesh and agricultural products were added to it. And, of course, as groups of men moved into cold and snow-bound areas, they relied more and more, sometimes exclusively, on fish and meat. But there are many persons dwelling in warmer, greener countries who live on plants, cereals and nuts alone, and who do without not only fish and flesh, but also without milk or milk products of any kind whatever. Today with better control of nature, men are changing their food habits in many cold areas, eating more vegetables and fruits and certainly feeling the better for it.

At this point I want to relate some personal experiences which will not only bring home a point but also shed some interesting light on certain styles of living.

At one time, during long years of travel and sojourn through the vast Himalayas, I lived in a locality deep in the interior of its western ranges and remote from the plains. It lay on the Ganges; on the road leading to the river's source high in the glaciers. Uttarkashi, or North Benares, was then part of the territory in the mountains bordering southwestern Tibet belonging to the native state of Tehri Garwahl, for the British had not as yet left India. The ancient dust road, trod from times immemorial by pioneers and pilgrims in search of land, adventure and solitude, led to the place which, at the time I am speaking of, could only be reached by foot or on horseback. The road was narrow and winding, running up and down along the mountain sides. It took nearly four days from the foot hills, climbing and descending through the slopes of the outer Himalayas and walking on an average of 20 miles a day, to get to the area. Being a mendicant pilgrim at the time, I made the journey on foot, carrying a small bundle of blankets, clothes and books on my back; a begging bowl and a water pot in one hand, and a long stick in the other. I got my food by begging.

Uttarkashi is a solitary retreat for a small colony of ascetics in a narrow gorge between steep mountain sides, peopled with forests of broad-leaf himalayan oak and tall resinous pines, through which the Ganges roars down in turbulent rapids on a bed strewn over with pebbles, rocks and boulders. The place was selected by ascetics in ancient times who wished to be near the holy Ganges yet far from the haunts of men and the distractions of society. The Ganges at Uttarkashi bends and flows northward in the reverse direction for a while, due to a geographical freak, as it does again at Benares far below in the plains. This is the reason why the place was called Uttarkashi or North Benares (Kashi) and regarded with such veneration.

The older ascetic settlements in the foot hills of the outer Himalayas, where the Ganges issues out of the mountain valleys into the north Indian plains, were at one time secluded and quiet, but with the coming of modern roads and railways they grew noisy and crowded, and were often frequented by charlatans. Today these places, where many old ashramas still exist, are as solitary, quiet and holy as Times Square in New York or Piccadilly Circus in London.

By the way, these are the areas where tourists and reporters from abroad generally congregate and gather impressions and materials for their observations on "secret" India. A few holy men are always on display in these places from dawn till dark for the benefit of such visitors.

Uttarkashi was then and is now a quiet place. We lived there in a number of small isolated thatched huts with mud walls and mud floors; some chose to live in mountain caves. We generally had two coarse blankets, one to spread on the floor, the other to cover ourselves with at night, for the place was at an elevation of 4000 odd feet, and the nights, even in summer, were cool while it snowed occasionally in winter. We had a few Sanskrit books rolled up in a piece of cloth or tucked away in a cloth bag which also served as a pillow at night. The huts were without windows and so low that we had to bend our bodies to get through the narrow entrance and avoid being hit by the door lintel. Our belongings amounted to a few books, a couple of pieces of cotton cloth, a couple of shirts, a waterpot, a begging bowl, two blankets, and sometimes a woolen pullover.

The place was austere and inhospitable in several other ways. The valley was so deep and narrow that even in summer the sun would rise above the eastern ranges after ten in the morning and go down behind the western mountains at four. Before the shadows which fell across us from the east could lift, the shadows from the west began to lengthen. The territory was wild and, being warm in the low valleys in summer, was infested with bugs, scorpions, monkeys and cobras, which could not be killed in deference to the non-violent principles strictly observed by the community there. Before entering our huts, especially after rains, we always took a good look inside to be sure that no scorpion or cobra had crept or crawled in. Cobras and scorpions were often seen and cases of stings and bites were not uncommon.

The monkeys, the rhesus variety in particular, were rather vicious, pillaging the fields and trees, or whatever they could lay their hands on. The newcoming ascetics, innocent of their ways, were their special victims. The monkeys could somehow size them up, follow them stealthily from behind and suddenly snatch away the bread from the begging bowl or out of their hands, scattering some on the road and scampering off with the rest. They would even grimace and threaten to make them give up either their food or the chase. Even the old settlers, for whom the monkeys had more respect, were wary and kept a sharp eye on their movements.

An uncanny atmosphere fell upon the place at nightfall. People would not step out of the door without a lamp and then only for an imperative reason. Wild animals prowled around. We could hear their noises; the low growls of wild dogs and panthers and the sharp cries of barking deer. The thunderous roar of the Ganges was more pronounced at night; our huts were only a few feet from the rapids, and the mountains rose sharp and sheer on both sides.

At times the reverberating roars of Bengal tigers rose in a crescendo, echoing and reechoing through the narrow and winding valleys. This would frighten the monkeys who chattered and moaned, shivering in fright in the tree tops. I heard, though I had not seen it myself, that sometimes the monkeys would drop down paralyzed by fear and become easy prey of the wild animals.

The black Himalayan bears would come down in large numbers from the upper reaches of the north as the first snows fell on the distant mountain heights at the beginning of fall. The bears descended in search of food, especially acorn, but sometimes invaded fields and homes too. They would climb up a large oak tree at dusk, settle themselves securely on a big and sturdy branch reclining against the trunk, break and gather a mass of foliage around them and eat the acorns patiently through the whole night. One could hear the intermittent snapping of twigs and branches and the rustle of leaves as they worked from evening till the small hours of the morning. At dawn they would retire to deep mountain crevices below, dark and shady places, where they slept throughout the day. But they were also active during the day if their hunger had not been appeased. I have seen, in other areas of the Himalayas, the entire crop of a big apple tree finished off during the course of a night. They were rather dangerous if they had cubs. After foraging for a while in one area they would move away to another, usually going south and reaching sometimes as far down as the plains. With the approach of spring they returned to the cooler regions of the north.

A few hamlets, composed of half a dozen or so households each, clustered and nestled in the mountains above, a few miles away. Wheat, barley and potatoes were grown on small terraces cut out of the mountain sides by the villagers who also owned a few cows and bulls. Some had a few fruit trees—apples, peaches, apricots or plums— and raised a few vegetables, small in quantity and limited in variety.

The villagers had a hard time making a living out of the fields, which they had further to protect from the depredations of monkeys and porcupines. Sometimes panthers and tigers killed their cows and calves.

Still the villagers were generous and hospitable. In earlier times the ascetics used to go to the villages to beg food, but later some businessmen, *sheths,* from the plains had built two alms houses a mile away from where we lived where food was given us in the morning. The houses, or *satras* as they are called, stood near the local temple of Shiva, and close by a tiny grocer's store, where the villagers would buy salt, molasses, pepper, matches, kerosene and a few other odd things. There was also a small post office, where mail and news came from the plains once a week on the back of a mail-runner, who walked nearly 15 miles a day.

This was sort of the downtown area of the place, inhabited by a dozen persons or so, who took care of the different establishments there. Once in a fortnight a barber came from some distant village, and we could have a complete shave free, head, face and all, if we so wished. This, also, was the gift of the almshouses.

However, I preferred to keep my hair and beard for a variety of reasons, the compelling one being that the country-made razor, which looked more like a kitchen knife, was applied to all and sundry with a little cold Ganges water to soften hair and whiskers, but without any soap or antiseptic.

After hours of morning meditation and a bath in the dangerous and icy rapids of the Ganges, cold from the fresh-melted snows above, we used to walk with our water pots and begging bowls to the alms houses, where we were each given four to six chapatis or flat round unleavened whole wheat bread, somewhat like the Mexican tortillas, and a large glass of watery lentil soup. We carried the bread in a plate made of leaves or in a piece of cloth, and the soup in the bowl. Twice a week we got a few diced potatoes made into a sort of a curry and not weighing more than six ounces which, however, tasted like a great delicacy. For drink we had the water from the Ganges which we used to purify by letting the sand and mud settle overnight in an earthen vessel or bucket. We subsisted on this food and drink for months.

I had of course read about vitamins and balanced diet but at the time I gave no thought to them. I was thinner and somewhat emaciated but I did not lack energy and, as I will recount later, I used to walk 10 to 15 miles a day or even more in the mountains on that kind of ration, going to the glacial source of the Ganges or the icy cave of Amarnath in distant Kashmir, at one time even scaling mountains fifteen thousand feet high and treading through miles of snow.

At Uttarkashi I often felt famished in the evening, and to allay the pangs of hunger I would save a piece of bread or two from the morning meal. As the bread would dry up quickly in that atmosphere and become quite stiff by evening, I used to moisten it with a little water to make it easier to swallow. We lived on the theory that food was not for pleasure but just to keep body and soul together; eating was somewhat like doing a Kantian duty.

On rare occasions, in the spring and summer, a sheth from the distant plains would brave the mountains with his retinue and visit us on horseback or in the dundees, i.e., coaches carried by porters, in order to acquire merit or to ease his conscience, troubled by methods of acquiring fortune. At such times he would bring a few pieces of cloth for us and also give a feast or *bhandara* for the hungry holy men —halwa, farina pudding, *puri* or thin puffed bread fried in melted butter, potato curry and maybe a few pickles and sweets from the plains.

To be honest, we generally looked forward to such visits. One afternoon, I vividly recall, as I was reading, sitting near the door of my hut to get the light, I overheard a conversation among my neighbors who said that a sheth had arrived the day before and was going to give a good feast for us. At its mention, to my surprise and embarrassing self-revelation, my heart jumped and began to pound wildly at my scrawny chest. I could not have dreamed before that food could stir such emotions.

However, these visits by the sheths were rare and only in the season; in the fall and winter hardly anybody came.

Not far from where we lived there was, in another colony, a young man who wanted to top others in austerity. He collected, by begging in the villages, a big hoard of potatoes after the crop had been freshly harvested. For six months he retired into a mountain cave and lived on these raw potatoes and nothing else. He looked healthy to me; his skin was clear and shiny, his movements quick and agile, and he was not thin. He was known because of his unusual diet as the "potato father."

There was also another person who deserves mention. He was formerly a great wrestler in the court of a maharajah but later decided to turn into an ascetic. He was ranked high in the community there because of his extreme austere practices including the observance of complete silence. He did not carry a begging bowl but had only a water pot. He would take the bread in his hand, soak it in soup, and eat it right there in front of the almshouses without carrying it back to the huts as we did. He used to get up at 1 o'clock in the morning and sit for meditation till late morning hours when it was time to go for the alms, for the houses remained open only for a short while around noon.

When I first saw him he had already been there a long time. He was big and strong. We were all under observation of one another. There were no secret sources of nourishment. Yet the erstwhile athlete, though he might have lost some of his earlier weight, was rotund and vigorous enough on a diet of bread, soup and potatoes.

The bread we ate was made from whole wheat grown locally with natural manure which was then ground fresh in the water mills. The air and the water were pure. But that is not all. I am sure that people crave more food and eat more from nervous tension and exhaustion, and also that they assimilate the nutrients less for the same reason. If your mind is well-ordered, organized and not distracted by the objects you have chosen to disregard, and further if it is not subconsciously preoccupied with repressed emotions; in other words, if you have made certain decisions with conviction so that your mind is restrained and calm, there is very little waste in the body and the need for nourishment is small.

In crowded and noisy cities where people are pressured to live a life not their own, where nerves are constantly excited, and passions and desires endlessly stimulated without being satisfied, those who do not have real convictions or higher values to control and direct them require an inordinate amount of food and stimulants. Still they feel tired because of the constant drain of nervous energy.

After a few months stay at Uttarkashi, I left with a couple of fellow pilgrims for the source of the Ganges in the glaciers on the borders of Tibet. The road ahead was more than a hundred miles long, skirting up and down the steep mountain sides and along the deep and winding Ganges Valley. We made 10 to 15 miles a day; we were climbing higher and had to find food and shelter for the night, long before it became dark. Five to ten miles apart there were wayside shops and sheds where pilgrims could stay overnight. Sometimes we slept on a bench on the open veranda of a shop. In between these rest houses were only wild stretches of forest where nobody lived.

Our road sometimes overhung high precipices at the foot of which, a thousand feet or more below, the Ganges with its swirling waters breaking to foam and spray against rocks and pebbles, looked like a strip of white ribbon. In spots the road skirting the cliffs was so narrow that two could not walk abreast. Sheep, mules and men had often slipped and hurtled down to death below.

As we moved up to the higher altitudes in the north, the crops and vegetation changed. Barley replaced wheat, the pines and the oaks gave way to tall Himalayan cedars (deodars), birches, firs and finally junipers, which grew sparsely on the craggy slopes.

After a few days march, we came to a place called Harshil where we found that a mighty landslide had recently destroyed almost the whole village. The debris of mud and sand was so great that the little apple orchard which stood near the Ganges bed, and which belonged to the State, lay buried several feet under it. The usual channel of the Ganges was blocked, the water flowed in a hundred streams in all directions, and at one point ran through a small house which had been a sort of state record office. There was no sign of the road for quite a distance, and we had to make a detour through high and difficult terrain to reach the road again far beyond the village.

At Harshil and also further below, we saw two white men in boots, with knapsacks on their back, marching up the mountains. It was an unusual sight but we thought they were some adventurous young Europeans. Much later we saw them again at Uttarkashi after our return from the source of the Ganges, and learned that they were prisoners of war who had escaped from the prison at Dehra Din in the plains and had been making for Tibet. They were caught near Harshil by the State forest-officer who had been informed by the

British. Tibet was only a few miles away from where they were captured.

Many years later I came to know that one of the two men was Harrar who wrote the book, SEVEN YEARS IN TIBET, but at the time we had no idea of it. Harrar escaped for the second time and reached Tibet safely. At Uttarkashi while being taken down, he and his companions stopped at our cottages where we had some food together. It was in the summer of 1945.

The last leg of the journey was from a village named Dharali, 13 miles from Gangotri, toward which we were heading. This place was at an elevation of 9000 ft. It was also a small trading post where Tibetans would come in the summer with yaks and sheep. The sheep and the yaks were protected by fierce-looking Tibetan mastiffs who had broad, spiked metal bands round their neck to protect them from the blows of leopards and tigers. So armored, two of these Tibetan hounds could fight and cripple any panther or tiger who would attack their charges. They were trained to bite a leg and crush it.

In winter the villagers went down with their cattle to the lower valleys further south or to the plains below, and the place would lie dead and empty under a thick cover of snow.

We reached Dharali late in the afternoon and found a small shed to shelter us for the night. Along the road were a few log cabins with roofs of slate, circled round a small square, where merchandise was brought and exchanged during the annual fair. The fair had already taken place so the place was deserted. But the cabins where the merchants had stayed were black and grimy with soot and smoke from their fires, and the wooden floors were laden with wool, dust and vermin, yak and sheep droppings and bits of greasy cloth. We managed to clean up the floor of one with a broom made of juniper twigs and spread our folded blankets upon it to retire for the night.

It was the night before the full moon. I had scarcely slept for a couple of hours when I awoke from cold and excitement and noticed the moonlight coming through the chinks of the door. I got up and went out with the blanket wrapped round me. The sight I saw has remained deeply engraven in my memory. In the still night the moon shone in the clear blue sky above the deep mountain valley in which the Ganges lay like a sheet of molten silver. The air was pure, rarefied and somewhat aromatic; the silence unimaginable. In the distance there was a mountain, one side of which was covered with snow from its base to the peak. It was a massive triangle of white, like the side of a vast pyramid, glistening and sparkling in the light. Dark shadows and the soft light of the moon dappled the landscape, the peaks and the ranges around. How long I watched in awe and wonder, enchanted, I don't recall. The spectacle with its stillness, beauty and mystery was like magic, ethereal and unearthly.

At early dawn next day, even before the first rays of the sun lighted up the mountain tops above and tipped with gold the silver grey peaks of snow in the distance, we started on our journey, for we had a long and difficult climb before us. Climbing is hard after the sun is up. Halfway along the road we had to cross over the Ganges from one mountain peak to another over a bridge of rope. We had already crossed and re-crossed the Ganges several times in our journey on bridges of ropes and wood, but never like this. The peaks faced each other over a deep and precipitous chasm about fifty feet wide, while the Ganges flowed swiftly on its rocky bed more than a thousand feet below, forming eddies. Four ropes, tied to wooden posts on each side, lay across the abyss — two above and two about four feet below. Small, thin pieces of wood were tied to the lower ropes on either ends to form a narrow walk, the upper ropes were to hold as one crossed. Only one could pass at a time and the bridge swung violently as we walked upon it, one after the other.

Many accidents had happened there before, and also many pilgrims had jumped to their death below stirred by foolish sentiments.

We reached Gangotri after a strenuous climb. I had only a few pieces of jaggery, a few chick peas and the cold water from a wayside spring to eat and drink. It was afternoon when we arrived. The Ganges begins its descent here from the snowy beds, or the matted locks of Shiva according to legend. The place is a steep valley with mountains around it at an altitude of nearly 13,000 ft. where it snows even in summer. In winter the place is uninhabitable, the snow lying 10 to 12 feet deep, blocking the road and burying everything under it. There is a small temple, a rest house for pilgrims for staying overnight and a few huts where ascetics live in the spring and summer.

In one of the cottages which had a sort of porch with a thatched roof we saw Krishnashrama, a naked ascetic, widely known for his holiness and austerity. He was seated in the meditative pose and had no clothes on him. In front of him lay a slowly smouldering log in a bed of ashes, which provided a little warmth. The place was cold, the air bleak and raw, and snow lay around. The sun did not shine long there, it remained mostly hidden behind the peaks. And as soon as the sun went down or if a little drifting cloud hid it for a while the temperature plummetted swiftly in that rarefied atmosphere; one felt as if someone was pouring down cold from above in buckets.

I noticed Krishnashrama carefully. He was a man of strong build, broad, tall and muscular. His rather dark body was lightly covered with ash, his eyes were bloodshot, his hair long and matted, and his skin rough and hard like the hide of a water buffalo. He did not talk but had an attendant disciple who had attached herself to him to serve him. Impressive though his practices were, the expression on his face and the atmosphere around him did not mean much to me.

On reaching Gangotri I had a dip in the ice cold water and then sat on the cold stone floor of the temple for meditation for a couple of hours or so. This was not a wise thing to do on an empty stomach and without enough clothes in those cold and bleak surroundings. I had to pay for it, but I will not tell that story at present.

Strong aromatic herbs grew around the place, which had been used since ancient times by indigenous doctors for their stimulating effect on heart, nerves and glands.

After three days of rather forced stay at Gangotri I came back to Uttarkashi, and in a few days started walking down to the plains in order to visit the icy cave of Amarnath in the distant Kashmir. On reaching the plains I took a train for Lahore, which is now in West Pakistan, and from there went by bus to Srinagar in Kashmir. At Srinagar I met a few fellow pilgrims, and we went together to Amarnath. We made the journey on foot from the last bus stop at Pahalgam. The journey on foot was not long, about 40 miles, but we had to cross snowy mountains 15,000 ft. high. On our way back we made the distance of 40 miles in one day. During this journey too we lived by begging. Our food was mostly the same; chapatis, lentils and sometimes potatoes.

I have digressed somewhat, but purposely from the topic of food to make a few points which I have already stated and which I need not repeat. But I would like to say another word or two on some related matters.

Yoga is often identified with asceticism. This notion I have sought to dispel in an earlier section. However, there is also a mistaken idea about asceticism in the West. Asceticism which is spiritual is not a kind of senseless and morbid self-torture. It is a self-discipline, like that of an athlete, to train and organize the mind. It is positive in its aim like the breaking in of a vicious horse. It is for self-mastery and self-conquest and not for self-destruction.

Extreme asceticism and asceticism for its own sake have been condemned by the great teachers of yoga. If one chooses to lead an ascetic life without being unmindful of his obligations, it is up to him. There is, however, nothing superior about it. Powers of will and endurance are impressive and worthy of praise; but sometimes it is a greater asceticism to live and work in the world after you have realized its shallowness and stupidities — to pursue life's nobler aims undeterred by all that makes existence tragic and absurd.

Life is to be lived, there is no virtue in laying waste to it. If any discipline hinders or represses its multiform and rich expression, that kind of discipline or asceticism has no meaning.

At the same time the nobler expressions of spirit demand control and direction. It is therefore true, as the great men of India have taught, that we need in the morning of our life the clear and perfect note of a spiritual ideal to fit us for the trials of later years and to save us from the perils of uncertain desires — from cheap cynicism and final defeat. I have profited in my life from the little disciplines I have imposed on myself. Having seen and known the opposite sides of life, the very orthodox and the ultra modern, and having lived in quite a variety of circumstances and under different conditions, I think I have learned to distinguish true values from false glamor, real purpose from senseless preoccupations.

We must master life and not be made its victims. Though I see the absurdity of many traditional views and practices dogmatically followed, yet I perceive clearly and appreciate all the more, in the surroundings of an affluent society and a scientific civilization, the profound spiritual truths of my Indian heritage.

To return to the subject of food and fasting, food should be diversified as far as possible. If one keeps to the following varieties of food generally one can be sure of a healthy diet. Fresh vegetables, including roots, stems, leaves and flowers, salads, fruits (especially of the season), seeds and whole cereals, fresh fish (boiled and broiled), vegetable oils, yogurt (less butter, cheese and cream) and a lemon a day.

People very often take to wrong food and other improper means to reduce or control weight. Weight should be controlled by proper diet (natural), exercise and fasting. It is injurious to take pills or to rely on artificial foods. I have seen quite a number of scientific people without common sense. While counting calories people forget that they have teeth and digestive organs which need exercise. The liquid and soft foods which dispense with chewing are harmful for teeth. A doctor in a well-known hospital in Manhattan once told me how a friend of his damaged his teeth by depending on soft artificial food for some length of time. Dieting without exercise is unhealthy.

Fasting for grown men is a very healthy practice, both for getting rid of the morbid materials from the body as well as for improving the functioning of the various organs. There is an old Indian medical saying to the effect that fasting is the supreme medicine. Full moon and new moon days are specially good for fasting, but people who work may find it difficult to observe them. They can fast on weekends or on holidays.

GENERAL REMARKS ABOUT YOGA EXERCISES

Yoga exercises are not competitive. Yoga insists that a man live a life of his own dedicated to his well-being and happiness. The exercises however can be combined with other systems of physical culture and sports.

The exercises are suited for all, especially for the needs of people past their youth. They can be done with benefit all through life.

The exercises are to be done slowly and deliberately with concentration. All jerky and bouncing movements should be avoided. The positions in the static postures are held for some time. In the beginning the postures should be held only as long as one does not feel great discomfort. It is not advisable to go beyond these points without instruction.

The exercises should be done in a warm room filled with fresh air. Avoid drafts.

The best time for doing the exercises is evening when the body limbers up naturally. The hour before lunch is also a good time. The exercises can be divided into 1) simple stretchings in standing position and breathings and 2) postures on the floor. The stretchings, breathings and meditation can be done in the morning, while the postures can be practiced in the evening before dinner. Wait half an hour after the exercises before eating.

It is a good practice to take a warm shower after the postures. Turn the shower from warm to cool gradually. After drying yourself with a large towel take another and have a dry friction bath with it.

To learn to do the exercises in the proper manner, sequence and spirit, it is necessary to have the help of an experienced teacher. It is best to have individual lessons. Individual needs and requirements are different and much is lost in character and spirit in group lessons. Those who cannot have a teacher can follow the exercises given below by carefully studying the instructions. Avoid hurry and proceed gently and slowly. Books will be more useful after one has studied with a teacher.

BREATHING — PRELIMINARY REMARKS

Most of the breathing exercises should be done in a sitting position, in the easy, the perfect or in the lotus posture. The spine should be erect and in line with the neck and the head. The chest should be a little forward to maintain the natural springlike curvature of the spine. Clothing should be loose and minimum. Better without it altogether.

It is good to do a few stretching and limbering exercises in a standing position before going on to the breathing exercises. This is especially important in winter.

For beginners it is advisable to do the abdominal breathing (breathing exercise No. 1) in a supine position with the legs crouched as shown in the picture. Since this posture is relaxing others may adopt this too.

Those who cannot sit in a yoga posture may sit in a chair or on their heels or stand for practicing some of the breathings. In all cases, however, the back should be held straight as noted before.

Breathing exercises should be done on an empty stomach before meals or a few hours (3-4) after large meals. One can do them shortly after a light breakfast.

Have plenty of fresh air in the room when you do them but

avoid drafts. It is wonderful to do them in the open in spring and summer.

While doing the breathings keep the mind concentrated on the movements you are practicing and the flow of breath.

Three Simple Preliminary Breathings

The first three breathings are meant to stretch the different areas of the lungs to their fullest capacity by localizing and concentrating the effort on a special set of muscles.

1.   Abdominal Breathing   (Lying on back with legs crouched or sitting in the easy posture).

Keep the body still and relaxed. First breathe out completely through the mouth. Afterward always breathe in and out through the nose.

After first having breathed out completely through the mouth breathe in through the nose pushing the abdomen out, without moving the chest. Breathe out right away through the nose and draw the abdomen in and pause without breath from five to seven seconds. Repeat ten to fifteen times.

This breathing is for the exercise of the diaphragm and for stretching the lower lobes of the lungs. Concentrate your attention on the movement of the abdomen and do not move the chest. See picture on next page.

2.   Ribcage Breathing   (Sitting or standing).

First breathe out completely through the mouth. Then as you breathe in through the nose expand the ribs as much as you can. Keep the abdomen flat or indrawn and avoid breathing with the

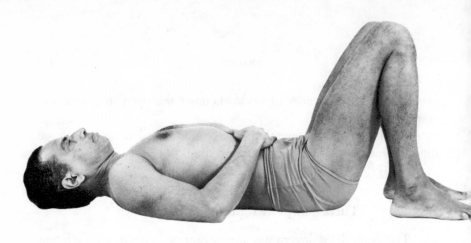

ABDOMINAL BREATHING

RIBCAGE BREATHING

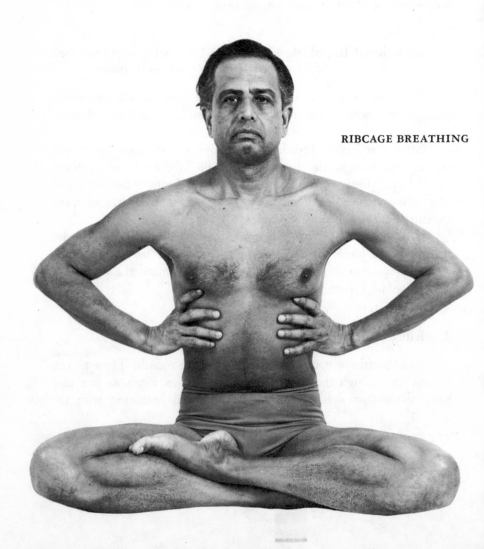

upper chest. To facilitate movement and concentration put your hands on your ribs as shown in the picture.

After breathing in hold the breath in for five to ten seconds and then breathe out. As you breathe out feel the ribs collapsing. Breathe in again without stopping and repeat ten times.

3. **Collarbone Breathing (Standing or sitting).**

The upper areas of the lungs, the apical areas, generally remain stagnant. Special effort is necessary to activate them.

This breathing also helps to build broad and square shoulders. Breathe out first through the mouth.

Keep your arms loose and relaxed. Imagine the ribcage is held in position by a metal vise. Keep the abdomen flat or indrawn.

As you breathe in through the nose concentrate your attention on the collarbone and shoulder area and feel that you are filling the upper areas of the lungs and that the hollow place above the collarbones is expanding. Take a couple of sniffs at the end moving the muscles in and around the neck region. Hold the air in for seven seconds. Repeat five to ten times.

This breathing and some others may cause a little dizziness in the beginning, but don't worry.

Complete Breathing (Sitting or standing).

1. **The best posture is the sitting posture, easy or lotus**

Keep the hands resting limp on the knees. Feel that the shoulders are loose and free.

First empty the lungs completely through the mouth. Then as you start breathing through the nose push the abdomen out slightly and then continue to breathe with the chest, while drawing the abdomen in, in the same process. Breathe in as deep as you can. The process should be continuous and not broken up—fluid, like the automatic transmission. It may be a little difficult in the beginning to follow the process correctly but practice will enable you to do it right in a short time.

Hold the breath in for ten to fifteen seconds and breathe out as slowly as you can. Breathe in again after a slight pause. Repeat ten times.

Later on, after you have learned to practice it well, make a little stop after exhalation too, say three to five seconds.

2. This is a variation of Complete Breathing 1 and is specially suitable for women.

Here you don't start with the abdomen as you breathe in, but start from the chest, and only at the end of breathing you push the abdomen out slightly. The rest is the same.

Regular practice of complete breathing will deepen your breath, cut down its rate, improve the heart and will have a profoundly beneficial effect on the nerves, the voice and the look.

Absolute Suspension (Lying or Sitting)

Lie as in the abdominal breathing position with hands against the thighs or sit, putting the hands against the knees.

Breathe out completely through the mouth and then draw the abdomen in as hard as you can so that you have a hollow below the ribs. At the same time contract the anal sphincters. Hold both contractions for five to ten seconds, then relax and take a deep breath through the nose. Repeat three to five times.

This breathing has excellent effect on many organs and nerves.

Bellows Breathing (Kapalabhati & Bhastrika)

Sit in the easy posture; lotus posture is recommended for those who can do it.

This is a breathing exercise of the abdominal type in which one breath follows another in quick succession. The chest remains un-expanded. The inhalation is passive while the exhalation is sudden and vigorous and is done by a quick contraction or an inward stroke of the abdominal muscles.

After each sudden and forceful expulsion of breath through abdominal contraction, the abdomen is relaxed and the inhalation takes place without effort. Combine this rapid breathing without pause as long as you can.

Make one or two such rounds in the beginning.

The breathing is unparalleled as an exercise for oxygenation. Its effect on nerves, upon circulatory and digestive systems and other anatomical parts is considerable. It has an important place in the daily physical culture program. There are several variations of this breathing, but they can be ignored by the general reader.

A Simple Pranayama

Sit in the easy or lotus posture. Place the back of the left hand on the left knee. Close the right nostril with the right thumb placing the index and the middle fingers on the bridge of the nose and keeping the ring and the little fingers free. Breathe in through the left nostril to the slow count of four, and then close the left nostril also with the little and the ring fingers. Hold the breath in for eight or, if you can, for twelve to sixteen counts, then open the right nostril and breathe out to the count of six or eight. Breathe in again through the right nostril, this time to the count of four, close both nostrils in the same way as before, hold the breath in for the same counts i.e., eight, twelve or sixteen. Breathe out through the left for six or eight counts. This makes one round.

Do three such rounds in the beginning.

Learn more about the proper method and meaning of pranayama from a teacher who has a grasp of the philosophy and technique of yoga meditation.

I want to add only one more breathing to this simple list. This is called Ujjayi and is performed as follows:

Ujjayi

Sit in the easy or lotus posture with the left hand resting on the left knee and the right hand on the right knee.

Expel all breath through the mouth. Contract the abdomen lightly and breathe in through the nose by partially closing the glottis but keeping the nostrils relaxed and open. A sobbing sound is produced by this breathing because of the partial closure of the glottis. Breathe in with the chest smoothly and continuously as long as you can, but keep the abdomen contracted. After a full inhalation close both nostrils in the manner described above in the simple pranayama and hold the breath as long as you easily can. Then breathe out through the left nostril keeping the glottis partially closed.

Repeat three times and increase to five later on.

Ujjayi is a most powerful chest exercise. There are variations of these breathings and other breathings which are for specialists only but are not recommended for the general reader. They can be learned properly from adepts.

Ujjayi Pranayama (Variation)

Ujjayi is one of the eight varieties of pranayama or breath control exercises mentioned in authoritative yoga books.

Sit in one of the meditative asanas. Hold the abdomen slightly contracted and take a deep breath through both nostrils by closing partially the glottis (the upper nasal aperture) at the junction of the throat and the nose. This will produce a sobbing sound, which should be continuous. The breathing should be smooth and uniform.

Close the glottis and do the jalandhara bandha (see later) i.e. press the chin against the throat and close both nostrils with your thumb and the little and ring fingers, placing the thumb on the right nostril and the others on the left.

Hold the breath as long as you easily can and releasing the lock and the closures breathe out easily and uniformly. Do it 6 to 10 times.

POSTURES

The posture movements of yoga are mainly spinal, abdominal and thoracio-diaphragmatic. The limb muscles are used to develop the most effective movements of the spinal and the abdominal areas. There are postures to aid the growth, efficiency and tone of the limb muscles, but they are supplementary to the main exercises.

Postures are both static and dynamic. In the static group, muscles are held in a state of sustained contraction for a desirable period of time, while in the dynamic phase the body is educated in motion along with posture and relaxation. The static posture patterns produce circulatory, respiratory, glandular and nervous changes which increase the vitality and efficiency of the body and create conditions most suitable for concentration, control and calmness of mind.

The postures are practically endless; their number has grown with the years. However, only a few of them are basic and important. There are several which are freaks in their nature.

Traditionally, there are 84 postures which are mentioned in the SHIVA SAMHITA, a later work belonging probably to the 17th century. But they are not all described in any one book. Of these postures about 33 are in general practice.

In the earliest hatha yoga text available today, the HATHA DIPIKA or HATHA YOGA PRADIPIKA, we find mention and description of 14 postures. YOGA PRADIPA mentions 21, GHERANDA SAMHITA 32, VISHVAKOSHA 32 and ANUBHAVA PRAKASHA 50. According to legend Mahadeva or Shiva, the great yogi, developed 8,400,000 postures from the observation and study of different animals.

The postures given here are more than enough for health, efficiency and vigor. They can be learned with patience and application. There are numerous persons who began yoga exercises after 40 or 50 years of age but who have mastered most of them. Those who begin earlier do wonderfully, if they are earnest, devoted and willing to take their time.

In India many people practice about 15 to 20 basic postures which are adequate to assure health and to reap the major benefits of the system of asanas. However, there are variations of several postures as well as some stretching and limbering movements which should be added to the static postures for allround education and exercise of the different muscles of the body.

POSTURES

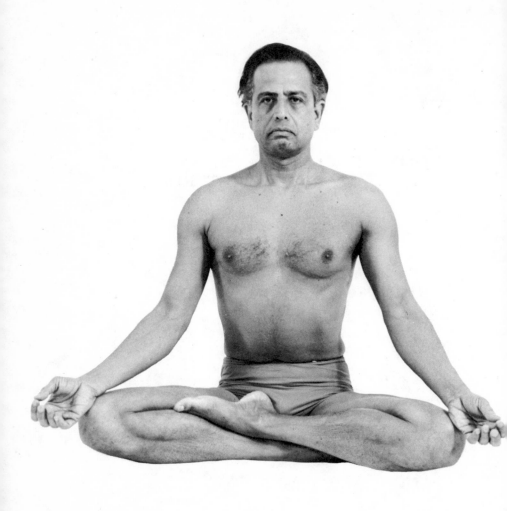

PERFECT POSTURE (Siddhasana)
(Easy posture for breathing and meditation)

Sit with both legs stretched. Bend the left leg at the knee and
bring the heel against the perineum or the opposite hip joint.

140

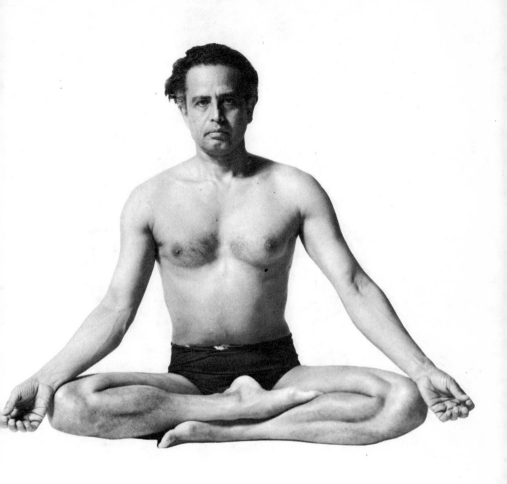

Next bend the right leg and put the right foot between the left calf and the left thigh.

Keep the arms resting loosely on the knees. The back should be kept straight — the head, the neck and the spine being in a line.

You can start with the right leg instead of the left if you find it more comfortable.

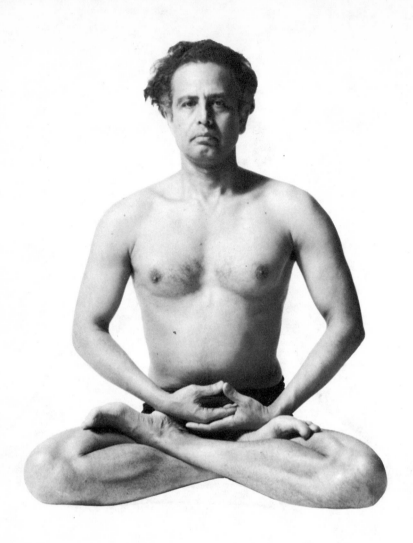

LOTUS POSTURE (Padmasana)

Sit with both legs stretched. Place the right foot on the left thigh, the heel touching the root of the left thigh with the sole upturned. Fold the other leg in the same manner. Adjust both heels so that they almost meet in front of the pelvic bones. Place the back of the left hand on the heels with the palm turned up, put the back of the right hand on the palm of the left in the same manner. You can also rest your hand on your knees loosely.

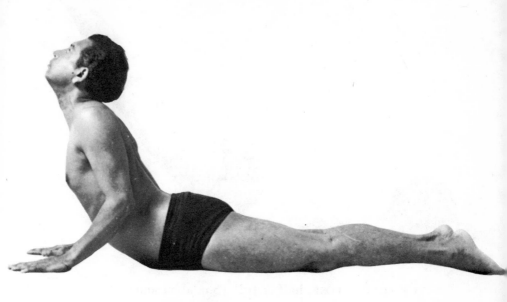

THE COBRA POSE (Bhujangasana)

Lie prone on the floor in a relaxed manner with the forehead touching the floor and the palms also resting on the floor lightly.

Raise the head bending the neck back as far as possible, throwing out the chin. With the head swung back, lift your chest by contracting the deep muscle of the back. After lifting the chest thus, work both with the back muscle and the hands; lift the lumbar area curving back so that you feel the whole pressure in the sacrum.

This is not a push-up. The spine should be bent or curved back step by step so that the pressure travels down the column gradually. The hips should remain on the floor.

Hold the posture for a few seconds and then lower the trunk step by step reversing the order followed in assuming the pose.

Breathe as you feel the need in the beginning. Later on do as the teacher tells you.

Practice five to seven times.

This is an excellent exercise for the spine, the deep muscles of the back, the spinal and sympathetic nerves and the abdomen.

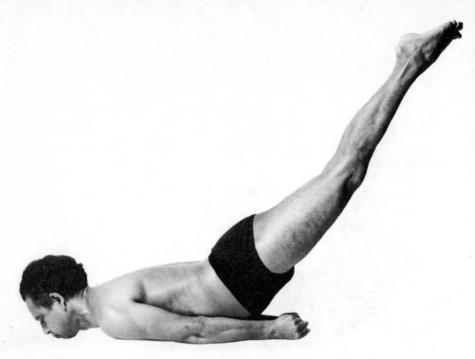

THE LOCUST POSE, half & full (Shalabhasana)

Lie prone on the floor with the shoulders and the chin resting on it, the arms stretched along the sides. Put the back of the hand on the floor and make fists which should be close to the thighs or just under them.

Lift one leg slowly but stiff without bending at the knee and making the greatest angle possible. Hold it up for a few seconds and then lower it slowly. Do the same with the other leg.

Take a deep breath before you lift the leg and hold it while lifting. Breathe out while lowering it.

Repeat about five times each.

Lie prone on the floor as before. Take a deep breath, stiffen the body and supporting yourself on the chest and the hands, lift the lower body as much as you can. The aim should be to lift the legs straight and raise the pelvic bones from the floor. Hold the position as long as you hold your breath, then lower the body, relax the muscles and exhale.

This asana is done with a sudden but smooth movement. It is a fine exercise for the hips, the abdomen, the pelvis and the lower back.

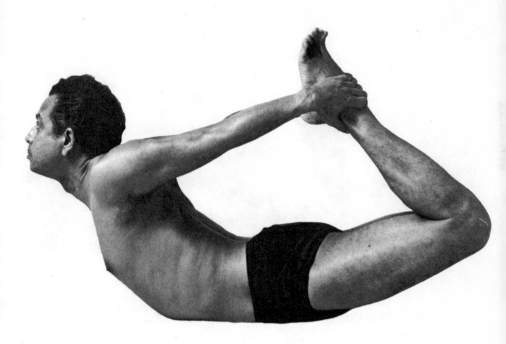

THE BOW POSE (Dhanurasana)

Lie prone on the floor with the chin resting on it. Bend your legs
at the knees. Grasp the ankles and raise your trunk as well as the
knees from the floor as high as you can. The whole body should
rest mostly on the abdomen and curve upward both ways like a bow.
Hold the pose for about five seconds then lower the chest and the
knees. Finally let go the hands and put them along the sides.
Breathing should flow normally.

Do it three to five times.

Apart from other advantages which it has in common with the
cobra and the locust poses, the bow pose stretches especially the
abdominal section and the muscles that flex the hip-joints.

145

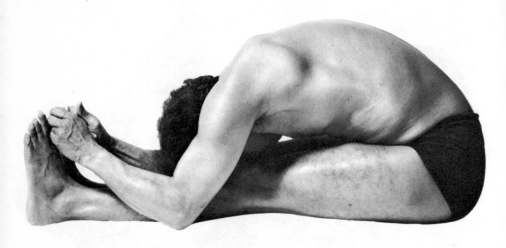

BACK-STRETCHING POSE (Pashchimottana Asana)

Lie on your back with the arms stretched on the floor over your head. Keep the legs close together. Take a deep breath, stiffen the body and sit up without lifting the legs.

Breathe out as you bend forward and down. Hold the ankles with both hands and keep the legs straight and bring the face down to the knees, bending the lumbo-sacral area and lowering the elbows to the floor.

Another way of doing the bending is to grab the toes with the fingers.

Don't be discouraged if you can't bend and get up properly at first. Try and maintain a steady but slow pull while bending. Don't bounce.

Repeat three to five times.

This is a very effective exercise for the back muscles of the body and the abdomen apart from its effect on the spine, especially the lumbo-sacral part of it.

146

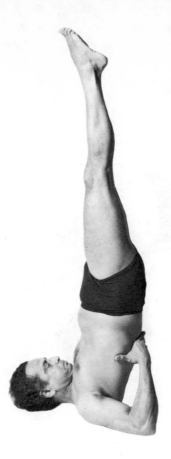

PANPHYSICAL POSE (Sarvangasana)

Lie on the floor relaxed, with arms stretched along the sides and palms touching the floor.

Raise your legs slowly through the hip joint and then taking the help of your arms and elbows raise the whole body with the legs thrown up. Support the upper back with your hands, make the body as much vertical as possible resting on the shoulders alone and press the chin against the chest.

Hold the position from a few seconds to begin with to a couple of minutes. Do it two or three times. Breathing is normal.

This exercise is recommended very much in yoga, principally for its effect on the whole organism through its action on the thyroid. It is excellent for the sex glands and the abdominal organs. It is also a good face-lift.

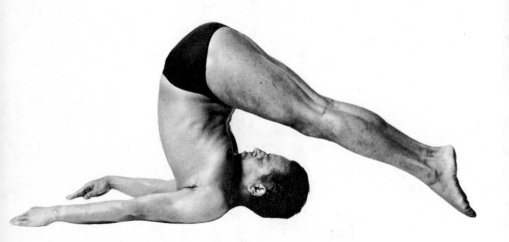

PLOW POSE (Halasana)

Lie on your back with arms stretched along the sides and the palms down.

Slowly raise the legs from the hip joint and then bring them over your head lifting the hip and the trunk. Gradually lower the toes to the floor, keeping the legs together. After holding thus for a while push the toes further and further away from the head till the pressure is felt in the dorsal area of the spine.

Stay for a couple of seconds in the beginning. No jerks or bouncing. Do it a couple of times.

It is regarded as a rejuvenating exercise, keeping the spine and the spinal nerves wonderfully healthy. It also strengthens the abdominal muscles and has a healthy effect on the thyroid and the abdominal organs.

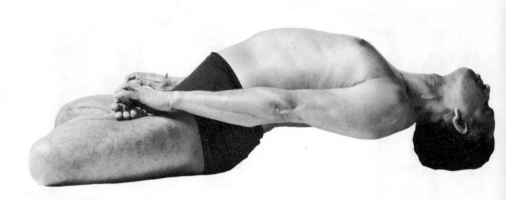

FISH POSTURE (Matsyasana)

Assume the lotus pose, lie on your back resting on your elbows and without lifting the knees. Then arch your back making a bridge with your seat and head. Next hook the toes with your forefingers.

This is a complimentary exercise to the panphysical pose and is recommended to reap its full benefits.

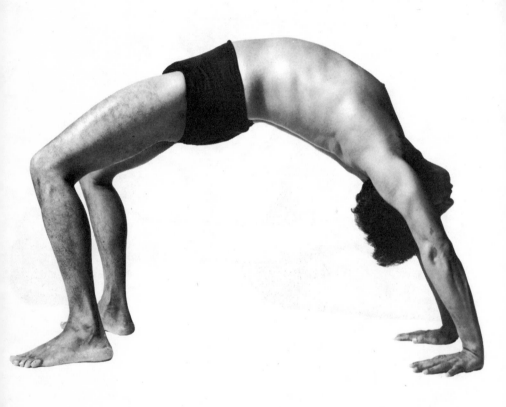

THE WHEEL (Chakrasana)

Lie on your back with the legs bent and the feet apart but close to the body. Bend your arms, putting the palms on the floor near the shoulders with the fingers pointing to them. Now raise your body like a bridge, resting it on the feet and the palms.

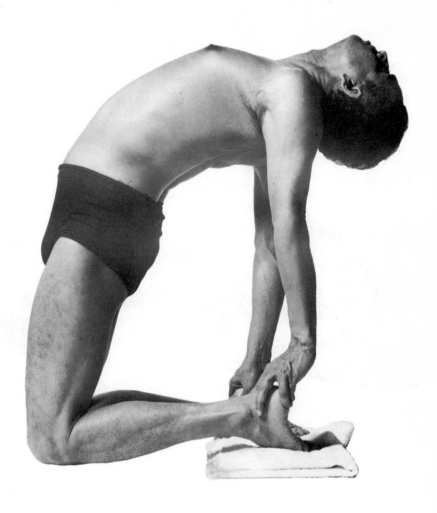

THE CAMEL POSE (Ushtrasana)

Stand on your knees, bend back keeping the thighs straight and hold the ankles with both hands. Lower your head as much as you can, to the floor if possible, but don't sit on your heels. Return to original position.

Repeat two to three times.

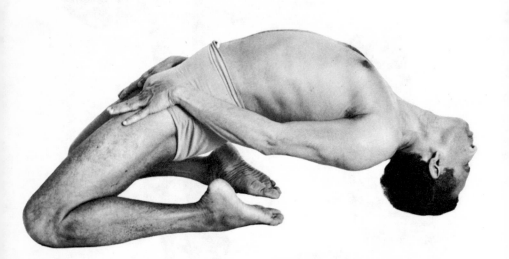

PELVIC POSE (Supta-Vajrasana)

Kneel on the floor with the legs apart, and gradually lower your seat to the floor between the feet. Lie on your back with the help of your elbows. Next put your palms on the thighs and arch your back as much as you can.

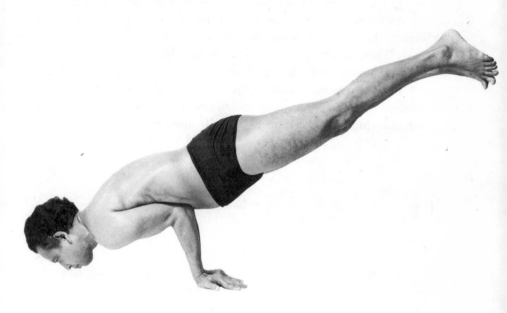

PEACOCK POSE (Mayurasana)

Kneel, put your palms together on the floor with the fingers pointing toward the legs. Support the lower ribs on your elbows. Lean forward and stretch your legs, slowly balance yourself by lifting the feet from the floor. By increasing the abdominal pressure this exercise promotes the health of the glands in the abdomen and also helps to reduce the fatty deposits there.

HEAD STAND (Shirshasana)

Interlock your fingers and put your hands on the floor so that your palms can form a cup to support the back of your head.

Put your head (front part) on the floor against the palms with the arms resting on the elbows and not making too wide an angle. Stretch the legs and bend the knees and bring them close to the chest. Then slowly jump up, just as you hop to ride a cycle, and balance yourself with the legs bent. Then slowly raise the legs up.

Practice against a wall in the beginning if you are alone, or let somebody else help you. Stay in position for a few seconds to begin with. Gradually increase up to 5 or 10 minutes.

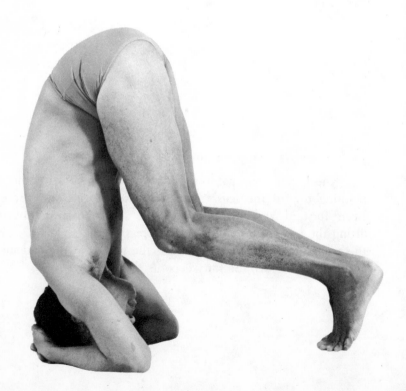

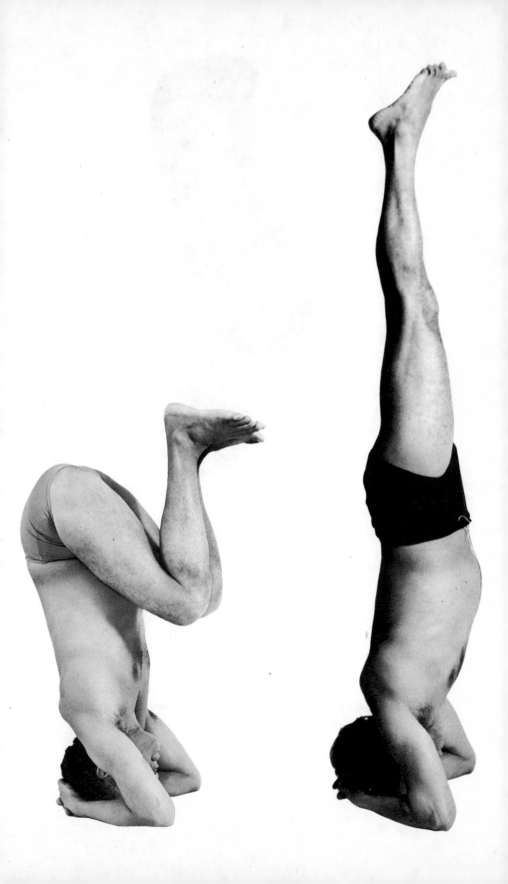

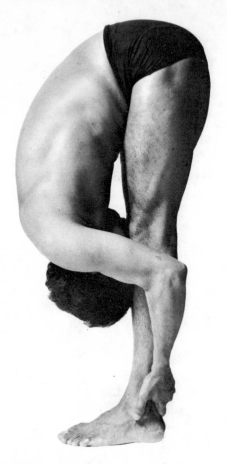

HEADKNEE BEND (Padahastasana)

Stand straight, raise arms and bend down touching the floor with your palms. Next grab your ankle and bring the face to the knees without bending them.

When you have mastered this, grab the toes with your fingers (the fore and the middle) and bring the face to the knees. Repeat three times. Stay down as long as you can. Don't bounce.

This exercise removes stiffness and tired feeling of the back. Further it firms and fashions the hips. It is a good exercise for women.

Breathe out as you bend down and breathe in as you stand up.

If you bend back with upraised hands before bending down, you get more results from the exercise.

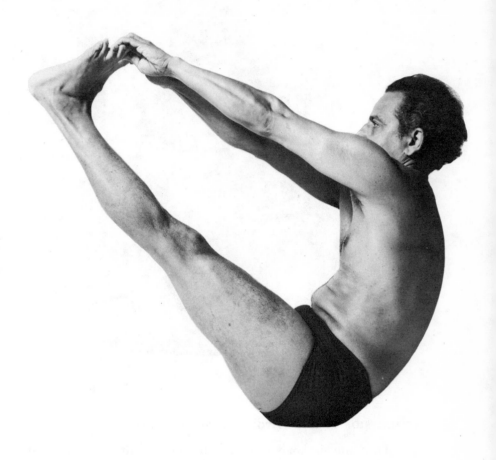

HIP STAND

Sit with the legs together on the floor. Lift the legs while bending backward and then grab the toes with your fingers. Stay up for a while.

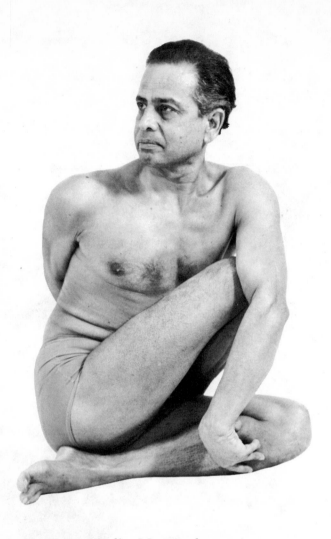

SPINAL SIDE TWISTS (Ardha Matsyendrasana)

There are six kinds of natural bendings of the spine; back and front, right and left, and right and left twists. It is important to practice these movements to maintain spinal health. Ardha Matsyendrasana bends and twists the spine on both sides and invigorates the nerve centers in the spine through muscular contraction and accelerated blood supply.

This posture is assumed in the following manner. Stretch your legs, and then bending the right leg press the right heel against the

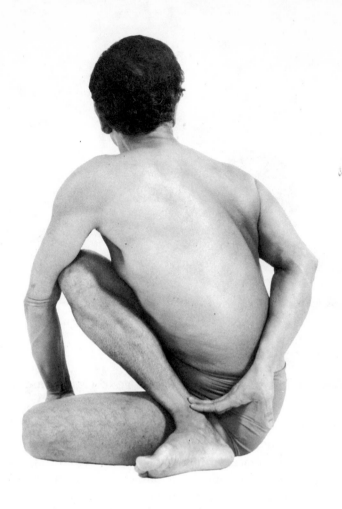

crotch. Sit on the right foot and bending the left leg take the left foot across the right thigh and put it on the floor. Next place the left knee under the right arm pit, while holding the right knee with your right hand. Then take the left arm behind the back and twisting the back, the head and the shoulders hold or touch the left ankle with your left hand. The head should turn left as far as possible and the chin should be above the left shoulder. The chest should be straight.

Hold the posture for a few seconds. Then do the reverse. Do it 2 or 3 times on each side. Breathing is normal.

159

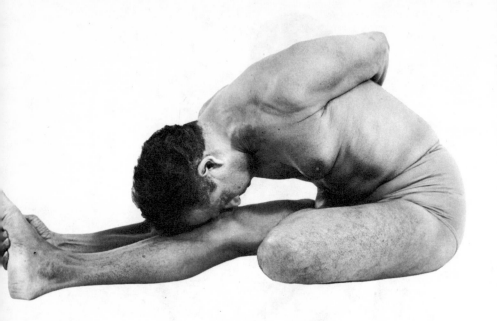

ALTERNATE LEG BEND or THE GREAT POSE (Mahamudra)

Mudras are static postures involving both contraction of a special set of muscles and pranayama or breath control. Mudras, properly done, are for higher control of bio-motor forces of the body, but some are also practiced in modified forms by those who do yoga for health reasons. Mahamudra is one of the important mudras. It is performed in the following manner.

Sit with your legs stretched. Next bend the left knee and place the left heel against the crotch with the help of your hands. Hold the right foot with both hands and contracting the abdomen slightly take a deep breath. After you have taken the breath pull the toes with both hands and bend your body down without bending the right knee. Then contract the anal sphincters, place the chin on throat or chest and lift the diaphragm up. Hold the breath for 10 seconds. Then release the contractions and resume the starting position. Reverse. Do it 3 to 6 times.

Mahamudra has important invigorating effects on the entire nervous system.

The above picture is a variant of Mahamudra.

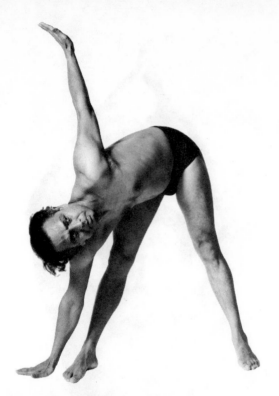

TRIANGLE POSE (Trikonasana)

Stand with your feet two or two and a half feet apart. Stretch out your arms straight from the shoulders in a line parallel with the floor. The legs should be straight and never bend at the knees.

Now bring the left arm down straight and touch either the toes of your left feet or the floor near it and keep the right arm in line with the left. Keep your gaze toward the right arm turning the face and neck toward the right shoulder.

Hold the posture for 5 to 10 seconds before returning to the standing position with the arms along your sides. Now do the reverse. Practice repeatedly for 3 to 6 times on each side.

There are many variations to it.

Trikonasana is an important spinal exercise and helps to relieve pain in the lumbar area which comes from weak muscles. Further, this exercise in particular has helped, to my knowledge, several individuals to add an inch or more to their height.

A few other postures are illustrated on following pages for which no description is necessary.

161

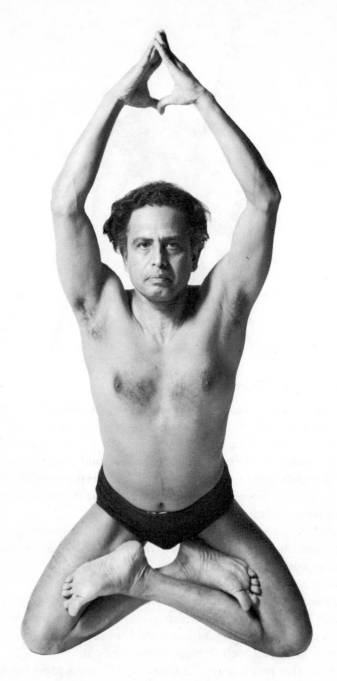

MOUNTAIN POSE (Parvatasana)

162

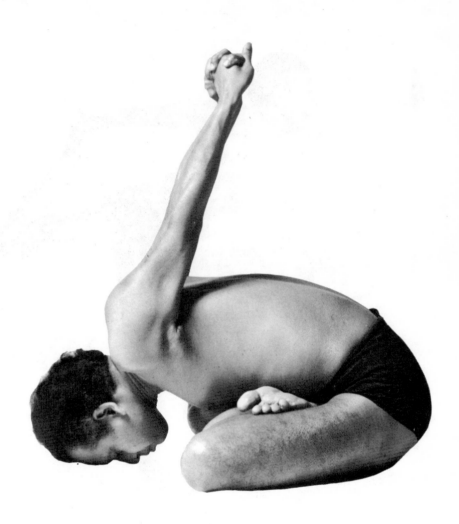

YOGA MUDRA

163

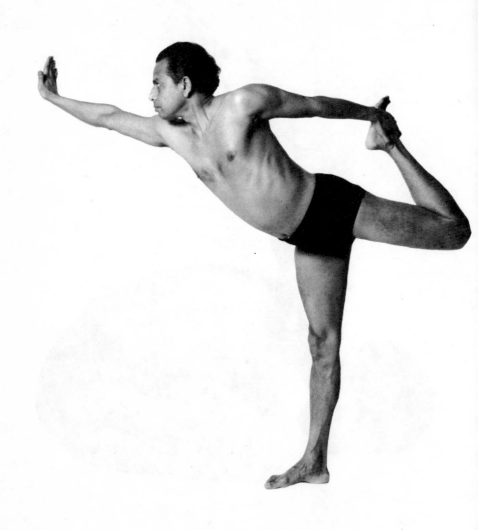

KING OF DANCER'S POSE (Natarajasana)

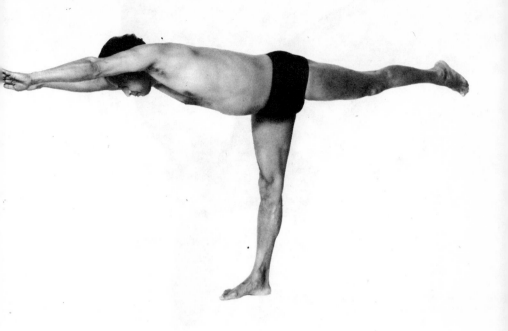

ONE LEG STAND (Ekapadasana)

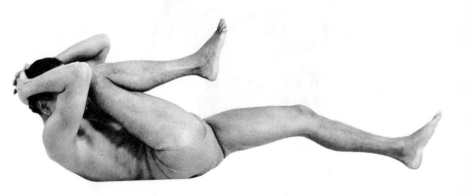

HEADKNEE BEND (Padahastasana)

165

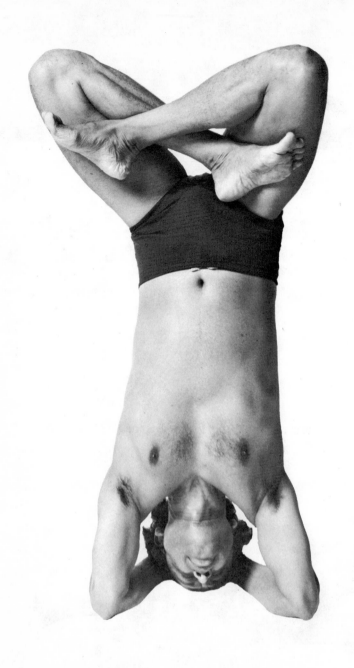

HEADSTAND IN BOUND LOTUS (Baddha Padmasana Shirshasana)

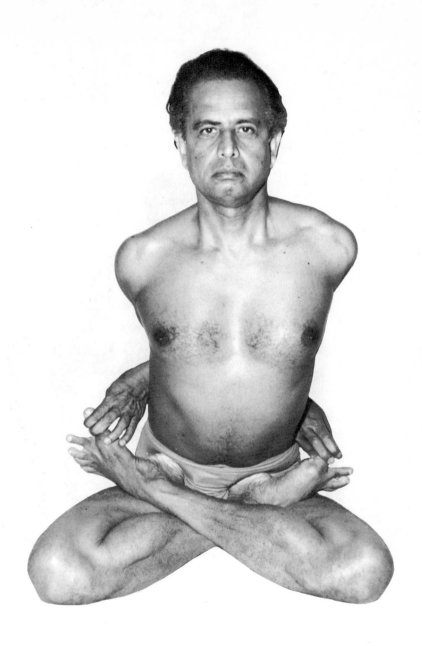

BOUND LOTUS POSE (Baddha Padmasana)

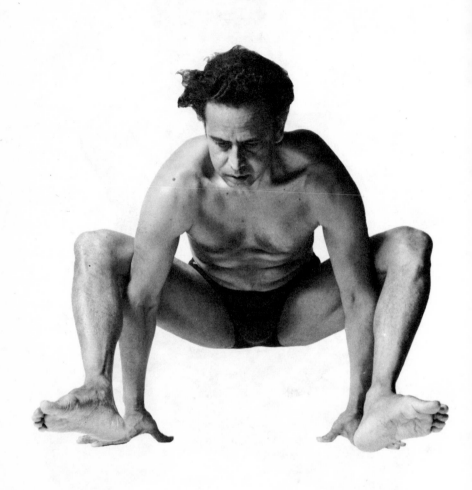

COCK POSE (Kukkutasana)

168

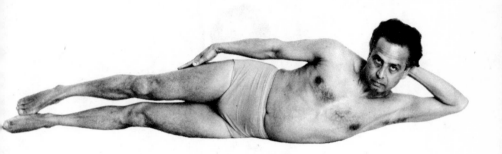

LATERAL SPINE POSTURE 1 (Uttitha Merudandasana)

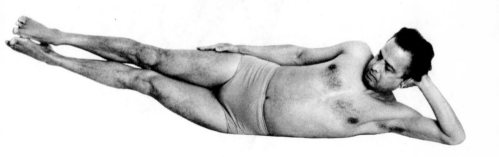

LATERAL SPINE POSTURE 2 (Uttitha Merudandasana)

169

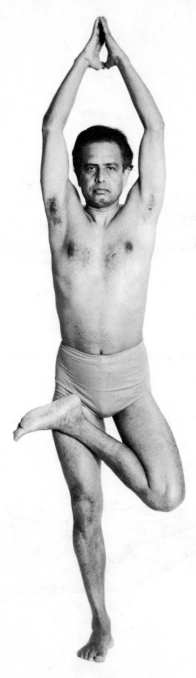

TREE POSE (Vrikshasana)

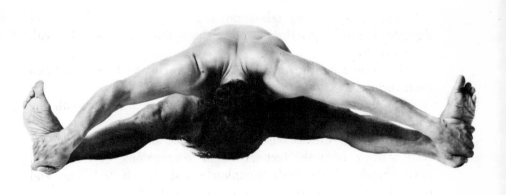

FORWARD HEAD-BEND (Bhunamanasana)

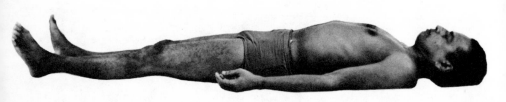

THE DEAD POSE (Shavasana)

This is a pose for relaxation and is practiced at the end of exercise. It can be practiced at other times also, independently, with great benefit.

Do it on a light mattress or a thick carpet spread on a hard and even surface.

Lie on your back with the arms resting on the floor with the palms up (see picture).

Close your eyes. Consciously relax the different parts of the body starting from the feet. Avoid all contractions. Feel that you have abandoned the body completely and that it lies limp and motionless and detached as it were from the mind.

Feel that you are apart from the body and that you are watching it passively. Observe your breath as it goes in and out without any attempt to control and regulate it.

After you have acquired some efficiency by practicing this over a period, try to breathe rhythmically.

Practice it from 10 to 20 minutes.

Shavasana has a profoundly calming effect on the nerves.

To relax fully right imagination, including the practice of detachment, is necessary. Imagination is the door to the realization of

truth. Imagination that takes us closer to truth denies our identification with the passing states of mind and asserts our pure, transcendent
Selfhood beyond all process.

There are, in each of us, profound depths of stillness, serenity
and wisdom, hidden under restless passions and desires, under our
fears, anxieties and illusions — depths we can reach through meditation and by letting go of our conditions.

After going through the preliminary steps of relaxation in the
dead pose imagine that you have left the world and all your daily
thoughts, cares and preoccupations behind you and that you are
retiring into the silent and luminous depths of Spirit, into its unbroken pure and tranquil Awareness. Practice every day and make
it a habit (see Meditation).

MUDRAS AND BANDHAS OR SPECIAL TECHNIQUES

The mudras are special techniques involving postures, contraction, breath regulation and concentration for attaining special
powers of control and perceptions. A list of twenty-five of them is
given in the GORAKSHA SAMHITA; the two more spectacular and widely
known of them being the *khechari* mudra and the *vajroli* mudra. In
the former, after the tongue has been lengthened by a series of
techniques its tip is turned inward and pressed against the palate and
the air passage. A person is thus enabled, along with other accessory
methods, to remain in a state of suspended animation for a long time.
Yogi Haridas remained buried underground for 40 days by doing
this mudra.

The vajroli mudra is a technique for sex control. By doing it
one can not only hold back completion of the sex act but also draw
up through the penis heavy fluids. I have not noticed higher and
enduring benefits flow from preoccupation with it.

A few of the simple mudras which are useful for health purposes
and are not difficult to practice have been described under the

postures. The rest can be ignored, being essential neither for health nor for spiritual reasons.

Bandhas are locks and contractions. The three chief bandhas are the uddiyana, the jalandhara and the mulabandha. The uddiyana will be described later.

Jalandharabandha

Jalandharabandha is the chin lock and is performed either in the lotus or the perfect pose.

Put your hands on the knees and press your chin firmly against the throat or on the chest a little below. This exerts an upward pull on the spine and the bunch of nerves inside and invigorates the nerve centers in the brain.

Practice it slowly and increase the pull gently. Don't hold too long in the beginning.

Mulabandha

Mulabandha is anal or pelvic contraction. It is performed in the perfect pose.

Press the perineum with one heel and stretch the other leg holding the toes or the ankle with both hands. Now contract the anal sphincters forcibly. Hold it for a few seconds and release. Alternate and practice 2 or 3 times. By acting directly on the nerve terminals of the anal sphincters, mulabandha works upon the central and sympathetic nerve systems.

THE PURIFYING OR CLEASING TECHNIQUES

In hatha yoga a group of six exercises are collectively known as shatkarmas or the six purifying acts. They are *dhauti, vasti, neti, nauli* or *lauliki, trataka* and *kapalabhati*. Of these dhauti and vasti are methods of washing and cleansing the entire alimentary system; neti is cleansing of the nasal passages, while nauli, trataka and kapalabhati are isolation of the abdominal recti muscles, fixed gazing, and short quick abdominal breathing, respectively.

As mentioned earlier, some of the cleansing methods are intricate and difficult and were originally recommended for persons with special health problems. They are designed for specialists who train for long suspension of breath etc. But there are some processes which will be found useful by nearly all.

Dhauti

Among the dhautis, literally washings, are the following:

1. Washing of the entire alimentary canal by drinking water and forcing it down and out through the intestines. This is called *varisara* and is learned after long practice.

2. Drinking in air into stomach by rolling up the tongue like the beak of a bird. This is called *vatasara*.

3. Pulling in the abdomen hard so that the navel almost touches the spine. This should be done after exhalation and in rapid succession. This is called *agnisara* or *vahnisara* and can be practiced either standing or sitting. While standing hold the hands against the thighs near the groin and bend forward slightly. This exercise is recommended. See uddiyana.

4. Drinking in air as in practice number 2 through the mouth and then expelling it through the intestines. This is known as *vahishkriti*.

Dental Care

Teeth can be well preserved and the mouth kept fresh and clean by following the simple practices mentioned below. These are generally recommended.

Mouth should be rinsed and teeth brushed not only mornings and nights on waking up and before retiring, but also after each meal.

For cleansing teeth besides brush and paste, the following method will be found effective in keeping them healthy and strong.

Have some kind of simple and fine powder, like a mixture of calcium carbonate, soda and salt (in proportions of 16:2:1:) and apply a little bit of it on the teeth with the moistened forefinger. Then rub and massage the teeth with the powder holding the teeth firmly between the thumb and the forefinger. Massage the gums also.

In India they use soft brushes made of twigs from certain trees, which are bitter and astringent. They are very good.

Also while cleansing the mouth in the morning scrape the tongue from the root with a tongue-scraper or with a brush and massage the root of the tongue with the three fingers, the fore, the middle and the ring. Then gargle with warm water. All this will keep the mouth clean and fresh and make the teeth whiter and stronger.

Several of my students have been saved a lot of time, trouble and expense by following these simple rules and have strengthened their teeth marvellously.

Tooth picks of wood or similar material should be occasionally used to clean the spaces between teeth where food particles often putrify and cause great damage.

Other Cleansings

There are methods of cleansing the oesophagus and the stomach with plant fibers and long strips of cheese cloth, but these are not advisable.

Vasti or Colonic Auto-lavage

Vasti is the practice of drawing in water through the rectum up into the transverse colon and then throwing it out. This and a few similar other practices which demand exceptional control over the abdominal recti muscles presuppose prior proficiency in nauli or abdomino-recti muscle control to be described later. However, for colonic cleansing and irrigation, a modern enema is good enough. Periodical enema helps to keep the intestines free from a large accumulation of poison-forming bacteria. Milk and milk products like yogurt, sour milk and buttermilk should be taken after an enema to replenish the intestines with healthy flora.

Neti

This is nasal cleansing and is done with the help of a piece of soft and waxed thread which is gently passed through one nostril and then drawn out through the mouth. Or, when sufficient skill has been attained, the thread can be passed through one nostril and drawn out through the other.

This is not too difficult a practice but is not generally advisable.

There is a simpler way of washing the nasal passage which can prove beneficial to many. This is by drawing in water through the nose and expelling it through the mouth. Fill the hollow of your palm with water and, putting your nose into it, close one nostril with a finger and draw in water through the other by a pumplike action in the throat. Expel the water through the mouth and alternate with the other nostril.

Use a little salt in tepid water in the beginning. Then gradually change to cool and cold water. After the nasal washings tilt your head in different directions back and forth and sidewise a few times to drain the water from the sinuses if any has got into them.

Nasal washing is a good hygenic practice, especially in cities with soot and dust-laden air. It has a stimulating effect on the brain, apart from keeping the nasal passages healthy and preventing cold and catarrh.

ABDOMINO-RECTI MUSCLE CONTROL

Nauli is isolation and rolling of the abdominal recti muscles. It is necessary to practice and learn uddiyana before doing nauli.

Stomach Lift (Uddiyana)

Uddiyana is an excellent exercise for the abdomen, the diaphragm and the ribs.

Uddiyana can be practiced in both sitting and standing positions. For beginners the standing position is more suitable.

Standing: Put your feet nearly a foot apart and bending forward slightly from the waist place the hands on your thighs near the

UDDIYANA

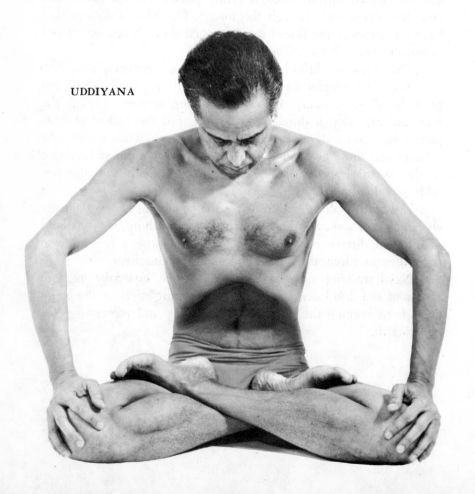

groins or on the knees. Empty your lungs with a full exhalation and, pressing your hands firmly against the thighs or knees, lift the diaphragm up aiming to touch the spine with your navel. When you find you cannot hold your breath out any longer, relax the neck and the shoulders, lower the ribs and take a full breath. Do this ten to fifteen times. You can also do this while holding your head firmly from behind with interlocked hands.

Further, while holding the breath out you can also relax and lift your abdomen and ribs repeatedly (flapping) as in mock breathing. This is a superior form of uddiyana and prepares the student for nauli. Uddiyana and nauli are best done in the morning on an empty stomach.

If you want to do uddiyana sitting, assume any of the postures for meditation, easy, perfect or lotus.

NAULI

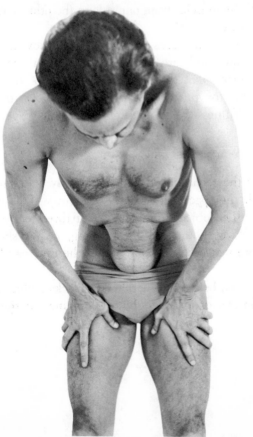

Isolation of Abdominal Recti (Nauli)

After you have acquired some proficiency in uddiyana try nauli. There are four varieties of it; central, right, left and rolling movements. Nauli is best done standing.

Assume the uddiyana position and bend the knees slightly. You can place your hands on the thighs. Exhale fully, draw the abdomen in and up, and pressing your hands against the thighs isolate and push forward the recti muscles. The two sides of the abdomen will remain soft and hollow while the middle portion should be hard and raised. Practice of flapping uddiyana will help to bring about this condition.

After you have practiced the central nauli, try the left and right naulis by manipulating the muscles separately. In doing these you have to lean on one side more, i.e., while isolating the right recti lean toward the right and while isolating the left lean to the left. Next try to roll the muscles from one side to the other with a swaying motion of the body.

Begin the different naulis with five or six movements each.

Uddiyana and nauli are regarded as excellent exercises for sex control and absorption of the external secretions of the gonads into the blood stream for purposes of reconstruction of the body and continued youthfulness. (See picture on previous page.)

TRATAKA

Trataka is the technique of gazing steadily at a suitable object on a level with the space between the eyebrows. This is done in a sitting position. The object should be about three feet away. At the beginning the gaze should not be too long, i.e., it should be discontinued before tears begin to flow. Later the time can be gradually increased.

The object can be a small marble or a black or blue circle of half an inch in diameter or a flickerless candle flame. At the end of the gazing, cup your closed eyes with both hands and feel darkness for some time.

Trataka is both an eye and concentration exercise. It should be done in the perfect pose or lotus pose.

KAPALABHATI

This is the quick abdominal breathing already described under breathing exercises.

GLANDS AND YOUTHFULNESS

The health and efficiency of the body, its youthfulness and capacity for resistance to disease and decay depend on the condition of the glands. While emotions and outlook play a large part in keeping the glands in a healthy state, there are physical factors which contribute toward it.

In many cases glands lose their efficiency prematurely. Various attempts have been made to maintain or revive their powers through transplantation, medication, injection or oral administration of glandular or other preparations. These methods have not achieved great success. Further, artificial stimulation has often led to their quick and permanent failure, besides often producing undesirable side effects.

Endocrine degeneration is not an isolated phenomenon but reflects imbalance of organic functionings due to lack of, among other things, muscular exercise, impurity of blood and its faulty circulation. Purity of blood and its proper circulation through exercise and right postures are essential for prolonged health and efficiency of the glands. Fasting, internal cleansings, and fresh, clean food which does not produce toxic substances are essential for maintaining the purity of blood. Overeating must be avoided. People have a notion that a two pound red steak will give them the vigor they want. But as experience shows this is a myth.

Many people lose their gonadal efficiency by wrong and uncontrolled thinking. The practice of detachment and conscious relaxation through meditation, cultivation of proper emotions, performance of yoga exercises to bring about accelerated blood circulation in the glands and decongestion in the pelvic regions will revive the efficiency of the glands.

There are static and dynamic exercises for endocrine development. The various special movements, breathing exercises and the inverted postures which have been given and illustrated before will help to restore and maintain the efficiency of the glands.

ORDER OF EXERCISES

Begin with a few stretching exercises in the standing position to limber and warm up. The following three are excellent for the purpose:

1. Stand upright with feet together and the arms hanging loose along the sides. Now holding the abdomen slightly contracted inhale slowly as you raise both arms straight and outward in line with the shoulders till you bring them up straight on two sides of the head making the palms face each other. Hold your breath and stretch your arms up straight alternately from the shoulders a few times, feeling the pull in the back all the way down to the hips and then drop them to the sides again while breathing out slowly. Do it 3 to 5 times.

2. Stand as in the first exercise and raise arms as before all the way up while taking a deep breath. Now hold your breath and join the thumbs together over the head, standing on your toes. Next pull yourself up as if you are elongating yourself by stretching and lifting the trunk from the waist. Then get down on your heels (still holding the breath) and bend from the waist to the right and then to the left without swaying the hips. Now straighten up, drop your arms to the sides and breathe out.

If you find it difficult to hold your breath all the time, take a breath when you need, but don't hurry and do the entire exercise slowly. Do this 3 to 5 times.

3. Stand up holding your hands together low behind back and inter-locking the fingers. Now take a deep breath and bend back from the waist stretching the arms and squeezing the shoulders. Bend the knees slightly also. Then bend forward down from the waist while breathing out and bringing the arms over the head as much as you can. Bring your head as close to the knees as possible but don't bend them. Resume normal position. Repeat 2 to 3 times. This exercise is excellent for relieving tension and pain in the shoulders.

After the above stretchings, to which you can add others, do the breathings and then the postures on the floor on a thick carpet. End with the dead pose.

The following basic exercises in the order given are good as a regular regimen. If you cannot do them all in the beginning, do whatever you can.

Add the other ones to the regular list as often as possible and have a break for a day or two every week.

Ordinarily 40 minutes of exercise a day will be adequate for the average person.

1. Simple stretch ups
2. Head knee bend
3. Perfect posture (or lotus) and the breathings with uddiyana
4. Cobra
5. Locust
6. Bow
7. Posterior stretch

8. Shoulder stand or Panphysical pose
9. Plow
10. Fish
11. Alternate leg bendings, Mahamudra
12. Wheel
13. Head stand
14. Dead pose

CONCLUDING REMARKS

I would like to make a few observations before closing this section on hatha yoga.

The exercises given are more than enough for all practical purposes. Those who want to go further and specialize will find the bibliography at the end of the book useful. To attain thoroughness and mastery over advanced techniques the need for a teacher and dedication to the subject are indispensable.

If you do the exercises described and illustrated above with care, patience and regularity you will realize their benefits and be able to develop from within yourself standards of judgment for estimating the worth and usefulness of many things written on the subject.

I have seen marvellous results flow from regular practice of yoga exercises. I have seen diseases, defects and conditions of different kinds like cysts, colitis, backaches, menstrual disorders, partial immobility from polio, arthritis, respiratory and cardiac troubles, overweight, insomnia and tensions relieved from the following of yoga disciplines. Many maintain and improve their health and appearance through the regular practice of yoga.

To reap results one needs seriousness, enthusiasm and application. But there are today, due to the general climate of public relationships, an increasing number of eternal shoppers who are too wary to trust and be serious about anything or pursue any worthy object steadily and earnestly. Such people do not go far in life in the realization of any of its true values or profound experiences, whether it is love, friendship or spiritual knowledge. They play safe and save themselves from both bad and good, remaining always indifferent.

IV
MEDITATION

IV

MEDITATION

RAJA YOGA

CLASSIFICATION AND DEFINITION OF TERMS

MEDITATION IS THE HEART of yoga practice. It is the supreme method of Self-knowledge. Meditation opens the door to subtle perceptions which change our convictions and character. Apart from its spiritual benefits meditation has a tonic effect on health. It calms emotions and strengthens nerves; and by acquainting us with the deeper workings of the mind, the *samskaras,* it enables us to attain self-mastery and serenity of spirit. Daily practice of meditation nourishes, like a wholesome meal, the roots of our personality making us healthier, stronger and happier.

All persons can and should practice meditation as part of their daily life, especially in a society where restless activity and endless distractions constantly draw them away from the basic truths and even the primary interests of life. Meditation gives the power to view life and its activity in perspective and with detachment so that we can judge things in their proper dimensions and true character. It gives poise and clarity of vision.

To practice meditation it is not necessary to have special beliefs or dogmas. All that is demanded is that a person have faith in his own self and truth and a sincere desire to find them through practice. However, it is essential before practicing meditation to have clear ideas about its nature, purpose and procedure.

First of all — the meaning of yogic meditation. Meditation in English means a kind of dwelling in thought on some feeling, idea or object. Here the mind is somewhat gathered and focused, but it is still diffused, discursive and revolving round its object, far from being completely quiet and motionless. Yogic meditation is perfect concentration where the mind is entirely steady and free from all fluctuations. Contemplation is a better word for this state since in its original Greek sense it meant the steady viewing of a single object like a flame without a flicker.

Such concentration requires long and unbroken practice and is not easily achieved. When we first begin, our mind wanders and we try to collect its movements within a limited area, taking as the object of our thought any image or idea which appeals to us. With steady and continuous practice the wanderings diminish and cease and the mind finally attains that perfect stillness which is called *samadhi* and which is the height of concentration.

The purpose of yogic meditation is to discover the Truth of our Self; in yogic parlance this is called *samadhi*. The object of meditation is Self. This type of meditation is therefore also called the practice of inwardness. The realm of existence that underlies or transcends the world of ordinary experience is infinite. As meditation deepens, layers and layers of this become open to our vision. The height of inwardness is achieved when we reach the state of Pure Awareness beyond all forms and mental operations.

Before turning to the various aids and accessories and methods of meditation, it will be useful to make clear a few technical terms.

Yogic concentration or contemplation has three stages according to its intensity. They are *dharana, dhyana* and *samadhi*. *Dharana* is the beginning of concentration. It is fixing the mind on some special centers of the body or on any other objects, external or internal. When the mind has ceased from wandering and dwells more or less steadily on one object, it is called dharana. Dharana deepens into *dhyana*, which is only an advanced form of the same process. In *dhyana* the mind flows continuously without a break toward its object, while in dharana the flow is not so continuous but intermittent like the dripping of water.

Finally, dhyana matures into samadhi which is complete absorption of the mind into its object or its perfect stillness without any object present to it at all. In dhyana one is aware of oneself as meditating; in samadhi the self-awareness is lost and the mind is completely one with the object, or is perfectly calm without an object. This is the technical distinction between dhyana and samadhi. Readers will recall the meanings of samadhi explained earlier.

Dhyana and samadhi are the two best known terms of yoga. They generally mean meditation and superconsciousness. The word zen or za-zen is a Japanese version of the Chinese word chan which is the Sanskrit word dyhana in its Chinese garb.

Zen Buddhism is a variety of yoga. Its roots are traceable through China to India. It arose in reaction to the endless intellectual bickering and fruitless logic-chopping which had become the supreme preoccupation of many Buddhist sects in China and Japan. It drew anew the spiritual seeker's attention to the fact that samadhi or satori is a suprarational experience and that meditation, not intellectual lucubration, is the means by which it is attained.

The three stages of concentration, namely, dharana, dhyana and samadhi, when they are repeatedly directed toward the different aspects of a single object with the object of gaining special knowledge and powers are known as *samyama*. Patanjali affirms that through mastery of samayama, one acquires supernormal powers and perceptions.

There is another practice which is akin to concentration and which is mentioned as a step prior to or concominant with concentration. This is called *pratyahara* or withdrawal. True *pratyahara* is withdrawal of the mind from sense objects. We are everyday aware of some kind of partial pratyahara, voluntary or involuntary. When our attention is absorbed by one sense object our mind is not receptive or not quite so receptive to impressions upon the other senses. Insane and hysterical persons as well as persons under hypnotic suggestion attain some kind of pratyahara when they become oblivious of their surroundings. They become so absorbed in their illusions and thoughts that they literally lose touch with reality. This, however, is not yogic pratyahara. Yogic pratyahara is completely under the control of the yogi. This is the power of voluntary withdrawal, the power of detaching attention completely from sense-objects and attaching it to some chosen internal object.

The best method of attaining pratyahara is to practice directing attention to one's mental occurrences exclusively by letting the mind drift and watching its flowing states as things apart from one's self. I shall deal with the subject more adequately later on.

Pratyahara is really the negative aspect of concentration. Pratyahara and concentration also follow from the practice of pranayama or breath-control. Such breath control again is not without the practice of some kind of concentration. The fact is that the various steps and processes of yoga are interrelated and interdependent. They do not come one after another in a precise logical order and sequence. They go together and help each other, though certain preliminary preparations are required before the practice of higher concentration. One cannot attain concentration without discipline of body and mind, nor can one properly govern body and mind without meditation. All the different yoga practices and steps are linked closely to one another.

PRACTICE

General Means

When we begin seriously practicing meditation we discover that gathering the mind from its ceaseless wanderings, fixing it on one object and making it steady as a flame without a flicker is quite a problem. In the sixth chapter of the Gita, Krishna declares that of all the spiritual seekers, the yogis who practice meditation are the best and urges Arjuna, the disciple, to become a yogi. To this Arjuna replies that the yoga of meditation which Krishna has described is extremely difficult to practice and that the mind is fickle, impetuous and obstinate, as difficult to control as the restless wind. Krishna agrees that the mind is not easy to subdue but assures Arjuna that it is brought under control through practice and detachment.

Traditionally these two, practice (*abhyasa*) and detachment (*vairagya*) are given as the general means of attaining samadhi or perfect stillness of mind. Practice means the practice of concentration and also of other aids and accessories of meditation. To attain sucess in meditation the practice should be long, continuous and uninterrupted; further it should be done with faith and fervor. Practice includes, among other things, the practice of detachment as well.

Detachment is not cold aloofness from society and the world, nor is it physical renunciation. Detachment is a mature attitude of mind which does not look upon the world and its goods and pleasures as the supreme goal of life but recognizes that life's fulfilment lies in the achievement of our true Manhood through freedom from the bondage of all illusions. Vairagya or yogic detachment is concern for the Supreme Good; it is neither selfish self-absorption nor indifference to neighbor or humanity. It is the repudiation of false gods and devotion to truth. It is idealism of the highest kind.

Practice of detachment is the cultivation of a realistic attitude toward life and the world. It is not the renunciaion of experience but of its bondage. Many who give up things externally cling fiercely to the little possessions they have, above all, to the little pride, the little ego, the little self. Detachment also includes the renunciation of the ideas of heaven. There are superior enjoyments and pleasures; the yogis do not deny them, but they all belong to the world of nature, the realm of maya. People who aspire after heaven are also chasing illusions and are in bondage. Detachment means, above all, detachment from the little self.

True vairagya or detachment is the sense of dissatisfaction with life as it is; it is the feeling of one who has done his part in the battle of life, who has tasted the world's gifts and prizes but has found them insufficient and has therefore turned away from them to something higher and worthier. Yoga is not an asylum for the maimed and the crippled, the weak and the defeated. Certainly, it helps many to recover confidence in life and conquer its prizes, but it gives no sanction to flight from life and world as intrinsically evil.

Detachment is not possible without faith in Self and therefore it always goes with *viveka* or discrimination. Viveka means discrimination between Self and non-self, between true identity and its superimposed conditions. Without viveka or discrimination there cannot be true detachment and without detachment there cannot be higher meditation.

Detachment gives us mastery over life. People who are victims of life cannot enjoy it; they are restless, they are in a hurry, they are dependent and insecure. We should learn to stand on our inner strength, the strength of spirit, the true dignity of man. The things of the world pass away; people who depend on them too much feel crushed and helpless when they are gone or clutch other illusions in an emotional rebound.

Yoga rules of conduct and self-discipline (*yama* and *niyama*) are for the purpose of attaining true detachment. The mind cannot be calm and balanced without self-discipline and self-direction. What law is to political liberty, ethics are to spiritual freedom. Ethical rules are like the banks of a river which guide its flow into the ocean where it becomes free. Without the steep banks, waters of the stream will not reach the goal but will be dispersed, dissipated and lost in the sands and soil of the landscape.

Ethical rules and ideals derive their true sanction and force from the dynamic and integral truth of man. Yoga repudiates all standards of conduct which go against the truth of man and bar the unfolding of his unique, as well as his universal nature. The truth of man is dynamic. The standards of today cannot be the guide posts of tomorrow. The ideals are there, fixed and inviolable as it were. They represent the highest truth of man. We all fall far short of them. But we must have the freedom of choice and we should approximate to them according to our understanding and ability. Principles which help us to grow into true manhood are the true rules of conduct; rules which suppress our personality are false.

Special Means

Beginners in yoga are often enchanted with the idea that they can storm the gates of samadhi by stilling their mind by a kind of tour de force without much prior preparation. There are others also who think that they can achieve the same object by changing the chemistry of their blood through drugs. This is not possible. The highest achievement of meditation, namely, the state of pure and objectless Awareness comes after long training and sustained practice of concentration with special objects and aids. It is true that there are instances of rare and gifted individuals who have stumbled upon superconscious experience suddenly as it were, but even in such cases one will discover, if one inquires, that the ground had been prepared before, though unnoticed, for such a consummation.

It is not possible to attain mastery over conscious thought without gaining knowledge and control of the subconscious. Samadhi, it will be recalled, is not mere stopping of conscious thinking or its suppression; it is the arrest and transcendance of all types of mental functionings. It demands long discipline and self-analysis to know and subdue the unconscious and the self-centered impulses of life.

Sometimes people confuse a dull, torpid or stupidly vacant, hypnotic state of mind with samadhi. But samadhi is no dark night of the mind; it is the full blaze of the noon of superconsciousness. People return from the experience of samadhi transformed; their ego has dissolved; they are humble yet strong; they are self-assured and without doubt. In the case of others who fall into a vacant state or a hysteric or hypnotic trance, the experience brings neither wisdom nor calmness nor any enhancement of their personality. They remain what they were before or probably get a little more confused.

This goes for drug experience too with some differences.

Generally it is essential for beginners in meditation to have a special object for concentration suited to the requirements of their nature and background. Competent yoga teachers help individuals in the choice of such objects and in the procedures of meditation. But broadly speaking the following objects and methods will be found helpful by most who would like to practice meditation seriously.

Practice of Self-Awareness

This is a practice which all intelligent and educated persons can follow with great benefit. It can be followed independently or as a prior aid before fixing the mind on any special object.

The practice is called *samprajanya* in Sanskrit.

The first and foremost obstacle to concentration is the self-forgetful tendency to float away helplessly on the stream of one's thought. The mind wanders. Under the influence of hope, fear and desire, the mind dwells on past experiences or future objects; it plans, resolves, imagines and dreams. The aim of this practice is to counteract the self-forgetful tendency of the mind and to arrest its wanderings by cultivating self-remembrance. This is done by holding the mind to the present, by observing over and over again like a spectator, with a part of the mind, what is happening right now in the body and the mind without thinking either of the past or the future. Let the mind drift. Watch the flow of thoughts and sensations as events and things apart from and outside of you; regard them as a procession of passengers entering the lighted room of consciousness and passing beyond into the darkness of outside. Don't let yourself be drawn away by the thoughts, desires, hopes or fears that come to mind. Don't push back or suppress anything that surfaces from the depths of the unconscious. Hold yourself apart from all occurrences and don't identify yourself with them.

In such observation you can also limit your attention to one type of object, say, just auditory sensations or tactile sensations or sensations of smell. If it is difficult to do this, observe whatever is present to mind but do not be drawn away to the past or the future objects. And if you find the mind has wandered away bring it back and fix it on the present.

This practice is highly prized by the yogis. It is the practice of recollection or remembrance. It purifies the mind by curing it of its restlessness and dullness. It ripens with continued and regular exercise into profound inwardness and serenity of spirit. In course of time the habit strengthens self-awareness so much that the mind ceases to wander and all outside objects are forgotten, i.e., perfect withdrawal takes place. In the degree that this self-awareness becomes finer and purer, to that degree the subtle truths of the spirit become manifest.

Meditation on the Divine Person, Ishwara

Most persons require a personal Ideal and depend on prayer and worship for making advance in spiritual life. Sri Krishna declares in the Gita that it is extremely difficult to meditate on the Impersonal Truth. It is therefore natural for the vast majority of men to worship a Personal Ideal. It is one of the best aids to spiritual growth.

The Divine Person is no other than our inmost self which is universal. In the beginning of spiritual life, we approach our own potential divinity as something other than and opposed to our little self. Devotion to and meditation on this Person make the mind calm and lead finally to the superconscious experience of samadhi and the perception of the Impersonal Truth of Self.

The Divine Person should be meditated on in the heart. This heart is not the physical heart but the area inside the chest where one experiences a feeling of happiness or delight when one is in love or otherwise very glad or joyful. It is also the area where one feels sadness or heaviness through fear and bereavement. One has to discover the place by tracing one's feelings. Our feelings are reflected in the heart area, but we cannot locate the area where thinking takes place. By meditating on the heart center we can easily reach the person who feels.

This heart area is the center of the physical "I" feeling or ego; the roots of our empirical personality lie here. The brain is the area of thought, but if thinking is voluntarily arrested for a while one feels that the "I" feeling is descending to the heart. After experiencing the subtle "I" feeling in the heart one can reach up to the brain by following its superfine flow and discover the center of the subtlest "I" sense there. Then the heart and the mind become one.

This heart area is not the solar plexus but above it in the spine.

For many it will be easier in the beginning to imagine a luminous smiling form, pleasant and tranquil, and meditate on it in the heart, thinking of oneself as part and parcel of it.

One should also at the same time repeat some name, preferably Om, and think of himself as calm, tranquil, steady and established in the form of the Divine Person.

Om is regarded by the yogis as the best sound symbol of the Divine Idea. Its repetition, inwardly, with the thought of what it stands for has a profound calming effect on the mind. Such inward repetition in a uniform and steady sequence controls the wanderings of the mind and concentrates it on the idea of the Divine.

At the beginning, the meditation may be a somewhat diffusive, and verbal dwelling on the form and ideas associated with it. Later when the mind has acquired some degree of steadiness, quiet and ability to dwell on the Divine Idea, one should imagine a translucent, white, luminous, infinite space in the heart that is pervaded by the omni-present Divine Intelligence. Then one should meditate upon his self as being interwoven and established in that Presence. While so meditating, one should feel without desire or thought, calm and tranquil.

The Mundaka Upanishad gives excellent hints on this meditation in the following verse:

"Om is the bow, the individual self is the arrow, the spirit is the target. It should be pierced with an unfaltering aim. One should then become one with it like the arrow that has penetrated the target."

This meditation is best practiced with the repetition of Om inwardly.

After some time one should give up all verbal thought of the Divine and identify oneself with the pure non-verbal feeling of delight alone. As the meditation deepens one goes beyond all forms and ego sense and becomes finally established in the Pure Awareness of Spirit.

The repetition of Om is called *pranava japa* and is done inwardly. Better and swifter results are gained by synchronizing its repetition with rhythms of breathing.

Patanjali mentions that the various obstructions to yoga like disease, dullness of mind, doubt, forgetfulness, laziness, distractions, hallucinations, false perceptions and unsteadiness are removed by meditation on the Divine Person.

There are many who have poor understanding of religion and declaim against the use of forms and images in worship. Wise men do not ridicule or condemn any aid or practice which helps an individual to advance in spiritual life. People need concrete aids and imaginations. Symbols are not idols.

Those who decry against forms and images are as idolatrous as any. They have signs and rituals, books and laws without which they cannot think of religion. Their ideas of God are vague and empty concepts. If they can pray to and worship such a vague conception of personality and hope to be heard, what's wrong with those who have a little more concrete imagination and who do not dogmatize about their notions of the Divine?

Meditation on the Divine Ruler is meditation on a higher truth than we are aware of. Man's normal feeling and attitude about his self and environment are false because our ego and will are not independent and free centers of action but are creations and puppets of cosmic forces which govern them. Yet this personal position of man is the right attitude so long as he has not perfected his individuality and distinguished himself clearly from the subconscious and preconscious mass-existence.

But the hold of this separatist, individualistic and aggressive stage of development on our consciousness has to be shaken off by realistic thought and practice if our child-soul is to reach the level of unity and universality which is the superior truth of life. The higher truth is the truth of our own Self though it seems so unlike, so remote and so contradictory and, therefore, so frightening to our little existence.

This is the truth behind the prescription and practice of humility and resignation which are the virtues of a hero and not the postures of an imbecile. Spiritual resignation is not the folding of arms and flight from battle but striving our best without worrying about results and remembering the higher power governing all happenings.

Sri Krishna says in the Gita that the Divine Ruler dwells in the hearts of all beings and moves them by His power like puppets mounted on a machine. The Divine Ruler is our inmost Self.

The Cosmic Person as Universal Power and Reason in history is the highest manifestation of the Impersonal Beyond. And though He is in the realm of maya, meditation on Him takes us beyond the bondage of maya.

Imagination is the door to Truth. But Truth should not be limited by any conception, nor should beliefs turn into dogmas. Man wants to measure the ocean of Truth with the cup of his mind. But Truth silences all talk. As long as man talks he is practical and struggling for Truth but far away from it.

PRANAYAMA

Pranayama is a distinctive feature of yoga. It literally means control of *prana*. *Prana* is an ancient Sanskrit term which means the energy of the universe that is expressed in different forms as mental, vital and physical activity. Prana also signifies life and breath which is the most obvious manifestation of the living process. Pranayama in yoga means regulation of breath with a view to controlling the life force, or the nervous energy, of the body.

Pranayama is one of the special methods of attaining samadhi. Yogic pranayama or regulation of breath is always practiced with

dhyana or meditation. Without dhyana there can be no proper pranayama. THE MAHABHARATA declares that if one practices pranayama
without dhyana one is apt to become more restless and nervous. Of
course this is said in regard to the difficult and strenuous breath control practices, which are often prolonged and which should not be
undertaken without preparation and understanding. But the simple
pranayama practices can be done by any intelligent individual. They
are beneficial for nerves and emotions. There is no danger in doing
them, though many popular writers keep on repeating, parrot-like,
solemn warnings about the harm they may do if practiced without
expert guidance.

Early in the history of yoga, the yogis noticed the close relationship between breathing and psychic conditions. Our emotional states,
our elation and depression, our joy and grief, our calmness and passion, our composure and conflicts are all reflected in our breathing.
Breathing slows down during quiet meditation and stops at the height
of concentration. They also noticed that through regulation of breath
it is possible to control physiological processes and to quiet the mind.
This is the origin of pranayama which was later developed into various
breathing exercises both for spiritual reasons and health.

Today physiological investigations have revealed that suspension
of breath by lowering the oxygen level in the blood, especially in the
blood vessels of the brain, produces a sense of relaxation and a certain
kind of withdrawal from outside. While this lends some sort of scientific support to the claims of pranayama as an aid to meditation,
changes in blood chemistry are not enough to produce yogic meditation and spiritual perception. Other preparations are necessary. Yoga
practices without doubt alter nerve currents and blood chemistry and
establish new neural paths, but these modifications are far too complex
and subtle for easy identification and simple enumeration, and are
induced integrally and psychologically through will and concentration.

It is also known today that the respiratory center, through its
connection with the vagus nerve, influences heart action and the
autonomic nervous system. Through pranayama it is possible to slow

down to a minimum all physiological activity including heart beats. These are well established facts.

Some simple forms of pranayama can be practiced by all. They are easy to do and are specially helpful for meditation. However, a few preliminaries are necessary prior to pranayama practice.

First, one should learn to sit in the proper manner. A special posture or asana is required for pranayama as well as for meditation, but particularly so in the case of pranayama. The ideal posture for many reasons is the lotus posture or the *padmasana*. But this is not essential. One can as well sit in the easy or perfect posture (*sukhasana* or *siddhasana*). The body should be held even and straight and relaxed, with the head, the neck and the back in a line. Eyes should be closed. The arms in the simple pranayamas may rest on the knees or on the lap with the hands one above the other. In the case of breathing alternately through the nostrils, the left hand should rest on the left knee with the palm up while the right should be used for closing the nostrils.

Second, it is also important that one learns a few simple breathing exercises before practicing pranayama.

The postures and the breathing exercises should be learned from a competent teacher or, in the absence of one, by following carefully the instructions given here.

The pranayamas mentioned in the earlier literature are simple but are to be accompanied in all cases with concentration.

Some Simple Pranayamas

1) Sit as mentioned in a quiet place on a soft seat on the floor with plenty of fresh air around. Wear clean clothes but as little and as light as possible. Better without any.

Breathe in slowly as much as you easily can and immediately after exhale very, very slowly as much as you can without pulling in the abdomen hard. Keep the body steady, still and relaxed and keep the mind empty and on the breath alone. After you have completed the exhalation suspend breathing as long as you can while keeping the body still and mind empty as before.

The attention can also be directed to the heart center during this pranayama.

Practice at least for a few minutes. This pranayama can be done for a long time and helps the mind to attain by stages the higher concentration.

A moderate and daily practice will make the mind tranquil.

2) Here is another simple pranayama but this is practiced with measure.

Breathe in slowly, keeping a count, and after a slight pause breathe out still more slowly with a larger count. Breathing out should always be more slow. Try the following counts in the beginning. 4:6, 6:9, 8:12, 12:18: Have a little stop also (no count) after breathing out.

Keep the mind empty and follow the movement of breath.

3) This pranayama is without count. Concentrate your attention in the heart center. As you inhale imagine that the breath is radiating from the heart to all the limbs and extremities of the body like a subtle and pleasant current. Breathe out very slowly and feel that the current is being withdrawn and concentrated in the heart again.

This practice purifies nerves, i.e., makes them restful, brings increased awareness to the whole body and produces a very pleasant feeling all over it.

After you have practiced this for a while stop at the end of each exhalation as long as you can and keep concentrating on the heart area, imagining that it is filled with a feeling of tangible delight as it were. Try to recall the feeling of happiness one experiences in the heart when in love, the feeling that comes from the remembrance of a beloved one. Do this as long as you can.

Later you can keep your attention on other areas and centers of the body. You can visualize the carotid artery which takes blood from the heart to the brain as a luminous stream. Or you can visualize a light on top of the brain.

Still there is another variation which you can try. While exhaling feel that all awareness is being withdrawn from the limbs and collected in the heart and then the gathered awareness is streaming up like a current from the heart to the brain. While breathing in, feel, as before, that the breath is radiating from the heart like a pleasant current to the peripheries of the body.

The heart area can also be conceived as the limitless, transparently blue sky or as an infinite translucent white luminous presence. The point at the center will be the heart center, and has to be located by tracing the reflected emotions to their place of origin as mentioned earlier.

4) Sit still and, keeping the chest unmoved, inhale and exhale by moving the abdomen only. It is a diaphragmatic breathing. Exhale very slowly and as long as you can. Breathe in noticing that the abdomen alone is expanding.

While breathing in and out in this fashion with the abdomen imagine a translucent luminous white space in the heart and feel that you are breathing into and also breathing out into the limitless space. Feel that the body has dissolved into space. Dwell on the feeling of empty luminous infinite space and on the heart as the center of that empty feeling.

After practicing this for some time, suspend breath after each exhalation as long as you can, meditating the while on the empty space.

You can also try another variation. Stop after each inhalation and imagine that the indrawn air has filled the empty space of the body like water filling a jar and has arrested all its restlessness and movement.

The above mentioned pranayamas can be done without any counts or with a simple measure. A simple method is to keep a count during the suspension only after either inhalation or exhalation. Stop say for eight seconds in the beginning and gradually increase. It is good to keep the counts by repeating Om inwardly.

5) Another simple but very helpful pranayama-meditation is the following: Sit quiet and imagine a blissful luminous feeling in the heart as mentioned before. Inhale and stop for a short while; exhale and stop a little longer. While exhaling imagine that you are deeply embracing the feeling of delight in the heart with the same effort with which you are squeezing the air out. After you have exhaled completely feel that you are holding the feeling of bliss in a firm embrace. Hold it for a while and then breathe in again. Continue for some time.

The breathing here also is diaphragmatic.

Pranayama has many varieties. It will be confusing and needless to mention more than a few. It is important in the beginning to learn to sit and breathe properly. Then start with a simple pranayama and a simple meditation. Stick to them for a while before you practice others. To get results you should be earnest and steadfast. Go about it with devotion and quiet seriousness; do not be hurried or lackadaisical. Dilettantes achieve nothing.

6) Finally, a couple more of pranayamas. These are later innovations but have become traditional and are most commonly practiced.

A. Sit still in the lotus or easy pose resting the back of your hand on the left knee. Keep your right hand free and place the two middle fingers on the bridge of the nose holding the other fingers loose for closing the nostrils.

Closing the right nostril with the right thumb, breathe in deeply and slowly through the left nostril. Then closing the left nostril with the little and ring fingers breathe out through the right. Without stopping, breathe in through the right and closing the right nostril again with the thumb, breathe out through

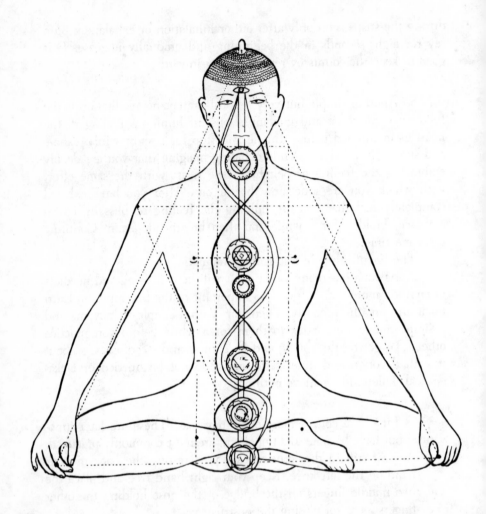

THE CHAKRAS OR LOTUSES OR CENTERS OF CONSCIOUSNESS

the left. This makes one round. Make at least three such rounds. Breathe in and out very slowly. Do not rush.

While inhaling imagine that a luminous current is flowing down along the spine from the top to its base and while breathing out feel that the current is flowing up the spine in the reverse manner. Repeat Om while breathing.

There is no count in the above pranayama but the next one is done with measure.

B. Sit holding the hands in the same way. Close the right nostril with the thumb and breathe in through the left to the count of four measures (two seconds). Close both nostrils and hold the breath in for eight measures, then breathe out through the right for six measures. Reverse the process breathing in through the right for four, holding the breath in for eight and letting it out through the left for six measures. Make at least three such rounds in the beginning and imagine the flow of currents up and down the spine as in the previous pranayama.

When you get used to doing it easily and without irregularity, change the measure and ratio. Begin with 4:16:8 and gradually increase, e.g., 6:12:9, 6:24:12, 8:16:12, 8:32:16, 16:64:32 and so on.

I have given enough for beginners. Those who will be ready to know and do more must make further enquiries.

THE KUNDALINI AND THE CHAKRAS

The Serpent Power and the Centers of Consciousness:

The aim of pranayama is to still the vital processes and control the nerve currents of the body for purposes of higher meditation. During this practice, yogis become aware of certain centers of consciousness in the body and also some special flow of nerve currents.

The centers of consciousness are called chakras and correspond to levels of awareness. The main channels of the neural currents are called *ida, pingala* and *shushumna*. The Kundalini literally means 'coiled up like a snake' and stands for the special nerve current which flows from the base of the spine to the top brain, stage by stage, piercing as it were, the different chakras or centers which are located along the length of the spine and also on top of it in the brain. The flow is felt only during deep meditation.

The Kundalini is so called i.e., coiled up, because it is asleep or inactive in ordinary individuals. It becomes active through meditation and spiritual practices and is felt to flow upward from the lowest center (*muladhara*), below the coccyx in the crotch where it is imagined as lying dormant ordinarily. The channel along which the Kundalini flows when awakened is called *shushumna*.

Meditation on the different centers or chakras is one of the great aids to success in pranayama and to spiritual knowledge.

The six centers, as mentioned earlier, lie along the shushumna which corresponds broadly to the spinal cord and extends from the lowest base below the genitals to the brain. The sympathetic chains which extend outside the spine on its two sides indicate the two nerve channels and currents called *ida* (left) and *pingala* (right). Shushumna contains two other nerve channels called *vajra* and *chitra*. All lie along and inside the spinal column.

Ordinarily, Kundalini is conceived as inactive and flowing downward. This power in its downward flow is the motor impulse along the spinal cord which initiates the various bodily movements. In other words the energy is occupied in worldly activities.

The spinal cord with its roots in the brain is regarded by the yogis as the chief center of the life-force (Prana). There are many centers of action in the spinal cord; there is also a center in the basal ganglia, the lower part of the brain, and there is the center of conscious thought in the cortical cells of the top brain.

The chakras or centers are not physical objects of flesh and tissue but subtle foci of consciousness. They are represented as lotuses of

different colors and petals for facility of meditation. Such representations have, of course, reasons behind them.

The first center is called the *muladhara,* the basal center, and is
located at the sex center below the genitals. The object of meditation
on this center is to collect the Kundalini power and make it flow
upward to the brain. Meditation on the centers is accompanied by a
strong imagination of the upward flow of Kundalini. The idea is to
bring it to the top brain and to concentrate on the Pure Spirit there.

The second center, called *svadhishthana,* is located a little above
the muladhara, between the navel and the coccyx. The third center
is *manipura;* it is inside the spine opposite the navel. Meditation on
this area and also on the solar plexus brings awareness of this chakra.
It is in this center that the reaction to sudden fear is felt—the feeling
in the pit of the stomach.

The heart center called the *anahata* chakra is the place where
we experience a feeling of delight and happiness from love and
affection. In meditation the center is to be thought of as located
inside the spinal column.

The heart center is very much mentioned in the Upanishads
and yoga books. The Upanishads call it the *dahara pundarika,* the
fine lotus, and also *Brahmabeshma,* the citadel of Brahman.

The heart center and the heart area are usually the best places for
meditation. Meditation on this center produces the realization of the
cosmic "I" sense. This meditation is called the meditation on the
Sorrowless Effulgence, because the experience gives rise to a supreme
feeling of joy and delight. This center is the center of physical or
empirical ego sense. The brain is the center of thought.

The fifth center is *vishuddha* and lies in the throat area. The
medulla oblongata is the place where shushumna joins the brain.
This is the center of vital force according to yoga. Above it between
the eyebrows is the two-petalled lotus, the *ajna* chakra. It is the center
of mind, the sensorium. The top brain is *sahasrara* or the thousand-
petalled lotus.

The aim of meditation on the centers is to collect the life force and nervous energy which are generally occupied in outward activity and awareness and make them flow upward along the shushumna to the top brain. This can be done also by concentrating on the thousand-petalled lotus in the top brain.

Through practice one acquires the skill to concentrate on the centers and feel the current along the spine. This practice is excellent for the health of body and mind. Meditation on these nerve centers improve their tone and function. Those who take it up seriously can feel it.

In hatha yoga, pranayama or arrest of the vital forces and the rousing of Kundalini along the shushumna are achieved through certain forceful (hatha means force or violence) practices of contraction (bandha) and other physiological methods called mudras. Such practice should of course go with spiritual motives and meditation. It is possible by such violent physical methods to gain control of the body and to control prana or the life force and attain the outward semblance of samadhi, but no spiritual illumination can be had by these means alone. Without the spiritual attitude and understanding and without meditation such practices lead to a state of suspended animation where the mind remains in a dark torpid state without illumination.

In the beginning of the last century there was in northern India a Hindu king who ruled over the last piece of independent territory in the subcontinent before the British swallowed it all up. His name was Ranjit Singh. He was a man of great courage and shrewdness.

Ranjit Singh was a man who was interested in many things including the doings of "holy men." To his court once came a famous hatha yogi named Haridas, who was reputed to have miraculous powers and who agreed to demonstrate some for a fee. He remained buried under ground for three months. After he had been raised from the grave, he was brought back to outer life and consciousness by his disciples who fomented his head with hot breads (thin flat Indian tortillas), applying them like hot pads. As soon as the yogi revived he asked the king, "Rex, do you believe me now?" and "Where is the money?"

This has been recorded by an English general who lived at the time in the court of Ranjit Singh. The English used to keep good watch on all the rulers and their doings. The Hindus generally did not preserve any accounts.

Haridas' case is a classic one. But there are other instances of many similar but not so spectacular feats tinged with commercialism. All this shows that the dramatic physical performances of hatha yoga do not necessarily indicate spirituality.

Prana can be controlled by other means too, and indirectly. Pranayama in the sense of complete control of all vital activity comes naturally to those whose mind becomes still and completely absorbed in meditation. As a matter of fact the breathing practices of pranayama originated from the observation of the immobile state of the body in samadhi.

Quiet meditation will lead to natural pranayama. But the pranayama practices are of value for meditation and for health.

Finally it must be emphasized once again that the channels shushumna, ida and pingala and the different chakras should not be conceived of in material terms and identified with the actual nerves and nerve centers or plexuses. They are subtle lines of direction of the flow of life-force or biomotor energy and foci of consciousness and should be meditated upon as such. It will be futile to seek their exact correspondence with physical nerves and ganglia as some have sought to do. Besides we do not know enough about the nerves and nerve chains and their intricate and intimate relationships and functions.

The literature on the subject of Kundalini and the chakras is large and confusing, especially the latter-day writings.

Originally in the Vedas, the *shushumna nadi* or conduit meant the channel of luminous awareness (the *brahmanadi*, the solar path from the heart to the brain) along the spine, the carotid artery and the pneumogastric nerve. In later times shushumna was mostly identified with the channel inside the spinal cord, especially the grey matter and the tube enclosed in the white tissues of the cord.

Practically speaking, all the nerves descending from the brain, both cranial and spinal, and the sympathetic chains, all of which extend through the spine and alongside of it to the area below the genitals carrying the afferent and efferent impulses are the seats of ida, pingala and shushumna. The actual currents and centers of yoga are discovered through meditation. They are subtle and they have locations but their relationship with the physical nerves and nerve centers are not quite clear.

MEDITATION ON FINE SENSE PERCEPTIONS

Meditation on fine sense perceptions is another special means of attaining samadhi. The fine sense perceptions come through concentration on special areas of sense organs. For example, concentration on the tip of the nose produces the perception of a pleasant scent unknown before. Concentration on the palate, above which lies the optic nerve, produces perception of unusual lights; concentration on the tip of the tongue produces perception of unusual taste; concentration on the middle of the tongue a wonderful feeling of touch; and concentration on the root of the tongue, which is connected and continuous with the ears and vocal cords, produces subtle perception of sound.

Also, if one gazes at the moon or any light or luminous object for a while and closes ones eyes one continues to see its image inside. Concentration on such images also produces special perceptions.

To obtain such perceptions it is necessary to practice concentration on the areas for a few days steadily in a quiet spot. Such perceptions make the mind inward and create faith in the higher truths. One must not get wrong ideas from such recommendations. The perceptions are not hallucinations, a thought to which the mind jumps quickly. They are perceptions of subtle nerve stimulations or nerve functions which remain unnoticeable to us ordinarily. They are not the products of wishes or expectations. They are noticed when the mind becomes quiet and objective. Such perceptions acquaint us with the subtle aspects of the sensible qualities.

MEDITATION ON THE DREAM EXPERIENCE
OR THE EXPERIENCE OF DEEP SLEEP

In many cases meditation on certain dream experiences helps to collect the mind and make it indrawn. In the dream our senses are inactive, there is a kind of natural withdrawal. There are persons whose minds are withdrawn easily from the environment if they are asked to concentrate on their dreams. For them such concentrations are helpful in producing samadhi.

Of course, you should not be carried away by associations while practicing concentration on the dream experiences. You should just steadily and vividly view the dream appearances.

You can also make the experience of dreamless sleep an object of meditation. Deep sleep is not loss of total awareness. There is a kind of vague indeterminate awareness in sleep. Try to recall such sleep experience without noticing anything around, without dreaming and without going to sleep. Try to recall sleep as a vague indeterminate awareness. There are a few individuals who find this not very difficult to do.

Meditation On Any Object You Like

Finally you can choose any object you like for meditation. But meditate on it inwardly. It can be the image or impression of any sense object.

Sometimes people find that if they try to meditate on a special object their mind is being constantly drawn to something else. In such cases one can meditate on that object steadily viewing it as the representation of a subtle spiritual truth. One should not allow the mind to wander but view the object steadily with a pleasant feeling of love or affection.

Sometimes some external object such as the steady flame of a candle, a shining surface or a black point are suggested for concentration. Persons of a hypnotic nature are often helped by this kind of concentration to achieve a degree of withdrawal and steadiness of mind. In such cases, if they do not lose their awareness or objectivity, they can use this method to make the mind still.

The viewing of such objects should be done steadily and without words, i.e., it should be a non-verbal awareness.

Such methods are not of a high order, however, and are not recommended for serious and intelligent students of yoga who should emphasize spiritual inwardness from the beginning.

A Simple Reflection

Another practice which may be called a sort of quasi meditation but which has a good spiritual effect can be followed by all who are not quite clear about the meaning and methods of meditation. This can be practiced without any special preliminaries of posture and breathing.

Before retiring for the night sit near the window putting out all the lights. Look out of it into the night and feel how the world has gone to sleep after the busy day, and then review in your mind all that you have done and gone through during the day, how much of it makes sense, the things for which you struggled or worried and rushed and hurried, how you acted and reacted, i.e., try to look at yourself objectively. Or you can imagine you have gone off to a far away star and are looking at the world below, dark and asleep. Think how millions of men daily struggle and fight, live for a while and then pass away, on a little planet spinning around a minor star. Look at the hopes and fears and joys and sorrows of little men.

Such thoughts and the very act of self-review will help you to see life in perspective and will gradually awaken the spiritual search. It will produce a more mature attitude toward the world and slacken the hold of foolish and false values on life.

The country, the mountain and the beach at night are the best places for such practice. The quiet dark night with its mystery helps to achieve an inward calm and detachment as we view things in the manner mentioned above.

MEDITATION AND HEALTH

Earlier in the section I stated that mediation has a tonic effect on nerves and health. I want to deal with the subject here somewhat specially.

Today the effects of thought and emotions on nerve functions and glandular secretions are well known. Most of the diseases in a well-nourished and opulent community are now traced to psychic disturbances. The most common killers and cripplers of today, namely, heart disease and arthritis are almost entirely of emotional origin.

The health, vitality and even the look and attractiveness of a grown up person in modern society are more a matter of mind than of anything else. Calm emotions, hope and dynamism in life keep persons healthy and vigorous. The kind of thoughts we think, mark and mold our face. Things do not remain hidden long. In later years conditions of the psyche, its hope and despair, its serenity and tension, all reveal themselves in health or disease, in comeliness or ugliness.

Meditation on Self, the practice of awareness of the fundamental Truth of our being, dissolves our tensions, fears and anxieties. It maintains the dynamism of the psyche and relieves us from that sense of inevitable discontent which goes with a materialistic and individualistic outlook. Feelings of true human warmth and idealism bring endearing qualities to face and look. Meditation gives undying hope and optimism, and the strength to bear lightly the joys and sorrows of life.

Apart from the indirect effects of meditation on health, our physical well-being and vitality can be beneficially affected directly through concentration. Through strong imagination and suggestion we can preserve and strengthen the pattern of nervous functions and physiological processes associated with the condition of health. Our thoughts are linked to certain changes in the brain and correspond to special neural paths. By steadily holding on to ideas of health and strength we can maintain those combinations and patterns. In case of sickness or disease strong imaginations of health help to rearrange the neural processes and functions into the healthy pattern which has been upset or disturbed. The body tends to follow the subtle changes which can be induced in the nerve centers and in the auto-nomic systems through the subtler powers of imagination.

Before going on to the practice of inner meditation it is beneficial to start with strong suggestions about the health and vitality of the different parts and organs of the body. Regard the body as the temple of Pure Spirit. Do not identify yourself with moods and feelings of weakness or helplessness. Deny all negative thoughts and sugges-tions.

One does not become perfect in a day. The more you practice with earnestness and consistency, the more you will become aware of its results. Don't panic and rush for pills under the impact of the slightest pain or suffering. Have faith in the hidden powers that lie asleep in the body and mind, and manifest them as much as you can. To take care of the body and attend to its needs in the right way are spiritual acts. Body can be both the prison and the temple of the Spirit.

To take proper care of the instruments of Spirit and to take pleasure and pride in them in the right way cannot be wrong as long as we remember where our true strength lies and as long as we do not set ourselves above others but recognize the same Spirit dwelling in every heart though hidden under covers of ignorance. Pride becomes foolish when we stand on the little passing things and qualities of nature and forget the essential truth of our Self.

Faith healing is a fact. But it is better to practice a little medita-tion on health and strength daily with a proper understanding of the underlying facts and principles involved and not wait till sickness strikes. You will be surprised at the amount of physical trouble you can avoid through this practice.

GENERAL REMARKS ON MEDITATION

In the foregoing section I have given the broad and general principles and practices of meditation. To be introduced properly to the subject of meditation, most people need personal instruction. But persons have to be ready for it. Without such readiness the instructions of the best teacher are wasted and of no avail.

However, there are some who are anxious to practice but lack opportunities for personal direction. For them some general hints will be useful as an introduction.

First, one should learn to sit in the manner mentioned before. But if you cannot assume that seat, sit in any other way which you can hold easily in a relaxed manner but keeping the back, the neck and the head in a line. You can, if you cannot do anything else, lie on your back, keeping the spine straight. This posture is not so good because people in this position tend to doze off into sleep and also because breathing is not so good and free.

Have a piece of thick rug on which you can sit on the floor. Keep it specially for meditation. Choose a quiet and clean spot and stick to it as much as you can. Have some flowers and incense before you.

You should practice regularly and daily, barring days when you are too tired or sick. It is good to keep to the same hours. If you keep the same seat and hours for a time you will find that the mind tends to get quiet and peaceful at the same hour and the same place. The place and the time recall by association quiet moods. This is the reason why places are called holy. The place where people think certain thoughts become charged with similar vibrations. There is an atmosphere everywhere — in churches, temples, schools, offices, clubs and night clubs — which affects|us.

Wear very light but clean, fresh clothes or even better, do without them.

Don't be in a hurry. As you sit for meditation imagine you are leaving behind the everyday world, closing the door of your mind to all outside things, and retiring into the vast, silent, luminous, inner realm of the Spirit.

Think of your body as the temple of the Spirit and as clean, pure, healthy and strong, part by part. Think that it is firm and flexible; pure and clean as a crystal; fresh, soft and supple like a fresh blown flower.

Next inhale and exhale slowly, thinking as you inhale that you are filling all your body with a wonderful luminous flow of health, strength and peace, and as you exhale feel you are throwing out all restlessness and impurities, all fears and anxieties. Do it a couple of times or more.

Then send out thoughts of love, peace and harmony to all those who are near and dear to you and to all the beings in the universe. Wish them happiness, health and Self-awakenment.

Pray for your own health of body and mind and for strength, light and wisdom. Pray to whomever you like, remembering that all are manifestations of the same Spirit and Principle, and that Infinite Power and Wisdom are behind all. Invoke that Power and Strength. The meaning and power of prayer will be known to you with practice.

Next do a few simple pranayamas as mentioned earlier.

After this, sit quietly for a while watching the mind. Let it drift, observe it like a child playing before you. But don't let yourself be dragged away by it in self-forgetfulness. Hold your attention to the present without planning, resolving, scheming or worrying. Do it for a few minutes.

Then begin the practice of meditation and concentration in any one of the ways mentioned before. Take up whatever suits you. Meditate as long as you can. Don't strain too much.

Offer a prayer again at the end of meditation and get up after taking a few deep breaths.

If the above is too much and complicated at the beginning do only as much as you can.

The best hours of meditation are early morning at sunrise, evening at sunset and the middle of the night. If you cannot observe these hours meditate when you get up from bed and when you retire or any other hour which you find available and convenient.

Do not meditate on a full stomach when blood goes to it to digest meals. It is a good practice to take a daily bath.

Some amount of physical exercise and activity are helpful for meditation.

After you have acquired proficiency in practice, you will not need rules. You will be able to meditate without such aids. Meditation in the sense of a calm, poised mind and quiet awareness will be continuous like a steady undercurrent flowing beneath all your activity and occupation.

DRUGS AND MENTAL HEALTH;
DRUG EXPERIENCE AND SAMADHI

There is quite an amount of interest today in a special group of drugs for their effect on the mind. There are drugs for tranquillity, drugs for inducing a state of euphoria and finally drugs which some claim produce what they conceive to be mystic experience or the feeling of internal freedom.

Drug experimentations have raised in many minds the possibilities of a novel but simple approach to the problem of mental health, character and even of some form of spiritual illumination.

The mind-body problem cannot be tackled with any degree of clarity and thoroughness without enough experience and without discarding the common sense notions about matter and mind. People tend to take a one-sided or superficial view.

Drugs affect the mind in many ways. They tranquillize and pacify. They can also derange the mind. Examination has revealed further that mental conditions are associated with certain chemical changes in the blood. From this it is tempting to jump to the conclusion that mental states are products of chemicals substances, and mental health can be restored through administration of drugs. There has always been a school of doctors who have believed in an exclusively physical and chemical approach to all kinds of sickness, believing mind to be a function of matter.

The problem is not so simple. The effects and side effects of drugs on the individual and his total personality are far from completely known. The tranquillity produced by the drugs is not the normal tranquillity. It seems to have been achieved at a price, by knocking out as it were some part of the mind or brain. People are restored from depression or turbulence to a kind of *blasé* normalcy and harmlessness. It seems a precious part of the personality, creative and self-regulative, has been lost.

This is not to say that the mild and occasional use of drugs to help patients in case of an intractable condition is reprehensible or inadvisable.

There is an intimate correlation between blood-chemistry and psychic states. From this it does not follow that mind and its states are a function of the brain or the product of chemical changes in the blood. Or that fundamental changes in character can be effected through drugs.

Facts contradict this, even if we ignore for the moment the philosophical premises underlying such assumptions. A healthy, active, balanced and cheerful person suddenly gets a mental shock from some bereavement, loss or other calamity. He breaks down and loses his mind. There was nothing wrong before in his blood chemistry. Rather the shock produces changes in the blood among other things, which are indications and effects rather than causes of the pathological condition.

The interrelationship between body and mind requires better understanding. Mind and body are two aspects of the same organism, of which mind is more subtle and fundamental. Physical and chemical arrangements of the body are expressions of mental factors; physical and chemical changes can hide, deflect or thwart mental operations. But mind still remains more powerful and its superior powers are realized in exceptional circumstances. People are healed of medically impossible and incurable diseases through faith and prayer. Most people are getting sick physically from purely psychic reasons. It is the mind which causes trouble to the body.

Psyche is not a function of the brain. Brain is material; but what is matter? The concept of matter has been on the anvil for some time, being fashioned and refashioned by new scientific discoveries and researches. Whatever it may finally turn out to be, it will certainly bear not a ghost of a resemblance to that conception which dominated nineteenth century physics and which lingers always in common-sense attitudes.

Drugs are useful in many cases; it is stupid to deny it. But the true healing power, which is in the organism, can and should be invoked without their aid. It is good to avoid drugs as far as possible and to rely with a little more patience on mental powers which are developed through exercise.

Drugs do not give us real health or true tranquillity. Mental peace and serenity depend on mental effort and pursuit of the dynamic truth of our being. Drugs often knock out that dynamic power through their side effects and leave us maimed.

Character or illumination likewise cannot be acquired through drugs. The experiences which the new drugs called hallucinogens produce are not true mystic experiences. These drugs in some cases give rise to unusually intense and sharp sense perceptions, dissolving the world into patterns of forces and also effecting some kind of release from the crude ego sense and the pressures and anxieties of everyday life. There is also a type of non-verbal, non-conceptual awareness of visions and impressions without a feeling of definite boundaries anywhere and a sense of intrinsic significance in the being of things, the every day practical motive having been inhibited.

All this sounds so mystical! But in point of fact this kind of drug experience has only a limited meaning. When the drug influence wears off only a memory is left, a faint one; nothing is changed in the fundamental attitude of the person to life and world. The old doubts, difficulties and problems remain.

The use of drugs of this kind and their effects have long been known. Sir Humphrey Davy, the inventor of the miners' lamp, once felt, under the influence of the laughing gas, that the whole material world became dissolved not only into vibrations but into ideas. In India *bhang* and *dhatura,* somewhat similar to marijuana, have long been used to produce pseudomystical feelings. American Indians who use special kinds of cactus fruit and mushrooms are not great examples of mystic wisdom and philosophical achievement like the Buddha and Socrates. Fortunately they lack the theoretical training to represent their flight into drug experience as mystic realizations and so mislead others.

In the fourth chapter of the Yoga Sutras, Patanjali mentions that some special powers of perception come, among other things, through the use of drugs. But they are not mystic experiences.

Besides the nature of the drug experiences is enough to show to a student of yoga that they are comparable, if at all, to the perceptions in the early stages of concentration, which are far from the realization of the supreme truth of samadhi.

True samadhi or mystic awareness is beyond all forms and determinations. There is no duality, no pattern, no process there; no distinction between the knower and the known. The result of such awareness is Illumination which changes the person's outlook completely. Mystics exude different qualities and speak in one voice. Samadhi cannot be reached by a chemical trick; it needs the preparation of our total personality and the integral discipline of character.

Recently many have gone completely out of their minds through use of LSD in their search of internal freedom. No wonder the drugs have been either banned or put under severe restrictions after psychologists and internal freedom seekers used them to carry on their experiments.

Drug experience is as far removed from mystic superconsciousness and yogic samadhi as are confused emotions and their silly
babblings from true love and its honest protestations.

Some day some one may discover a drug to keep a person in
love with another eternally. That will be terrible!

ETHICS: RULES OF CONDUCT

A philosophy which is a way of life and not an idle speculation
is based upon certain convictions born of the wisdom of experience;
it does not rest upon or draw its authority from mere probabilities
of reason. It has rules and standards of conduct to guide life to
wisdom and final fulfilment.

As will have been clear from what has gone before yoga is the
secret of living. It is only a methodized effort at achieving that altitude
of existence which life is subconsciously trying to attain through trial,
error and waste. Yoga is therefore not opposed to or apart from life.
Its rules are for guiding life and not for suppressing it.

Yoga ethics and rules of conduct derive ultimately from the
higher spiritual reality and goal of man, not from somewhere above,
nor from narrow social or utilitarian considerations. Their purpose is
to help man manifest the higher truth of Self by breaking through the
transitory mould of the ego in which his consciousness is imprisoned.
The rules are the laws of our growth.

The yoga ideal is the universal man for whom the unity of
existence is a concrete experience and in whom a perfect harmony
has been achieved between individual expression and universal
existence. Life and history hold this universal truth in their heart;
it is their secret dynamic.

The experience of the universal is also the feeling of love and
compassion for existence, the experience of the *Buddhahridaya,* the
heart of the Buddha, i.e., the heart of the enlightened man. Love is
knowledge; it is the summit of consciousness.

Yoga therefore proclaims that love or *ahimsa* is the one absolute ideal. Ahimsa is not only non-injury but also positive concern. Ahimsa has been declared to be the highest virtue or the ultimate truth of man or true manliness. All rules and standards of conduct have their ground and justification in this.

While the ideal is absolute and timeless, in actual life truth is manifold and dynamic. The child soul grows into the maturity of manhood by stages. Spiritual disciplines and ethical rules have to take into account the dynamic truth of life and the diversity of human nature. Rules which go against the truths of man's nature have neither meaning nor justification.

The dynamic truth of man and the diversity of human nature are recognized in the Upanishads and the Gita. We stand on different levels, and we have different natures. The truth of one is not the truth of another; the truth of today is not the truth of tomorrow. We have a common goal but we move toward it through diverse self-expression and at unequal speed. We must follow our own nature, otherwise we falsify ourselves. "It is better to die by following one's nature than to imitate another's virtue, however perfect."

Social rules, conventions and utilitarian motives are not the standards by which a yogi judges his conduct. His aim lies beyond.

Spirituality and ethics are not one and the same. Ethical conduct is essential for spiritual growth, but spiritual Self-realization demands more than ethical effort. Ethical rules and social standards are inadequate and crude transcriptions of spiritual truths. There is no perfect goodness in this world. All actions no matter how good have some evil in them judged by absolute standards. They are all shades of gray. "All actions are covered with some blemish like fire with smoke."

The absolute Good is a transcendental experience not attainable in the world of change and relations. It is there as an ideal for the world to copy in its relationships. But the world never becomes perfect. Men of evolved character cannot feel happy or rest content as long as there is hunger and disease, poverty and ignorance, suppression and exploitation, cruelty and violence in the world. They feel their obligation to all humanity and to all life. Their feelings are not confined to their own society, nation, race or religion. A sense of guilt oppresses the conscience of the universal man and urges him to exert effort toward relieving human misery and ignorance wherever they exist. Realization of the unity of existence is expressed in love, compassion, and charity. "He who looks upon everything with the same eye as he regards himself, whether in pleasure or pain, he is considered a perfect yogi."

Yoga disciplines are thus meant to take the student beyond the imperfect experience of ethical relationships to the transcendent experience of spiritual understanding, the source of ethical feelings and the goal of all effort. They are meant to free us from the domination of instincts, break the mould of the ego and thus attain the underlying and eternal Truth of non-dualistic consciousness. All thought and action which help to manifest the eternal truth of man in us is part of yoga. Anything which helps make us strong, free and universal is spiritual; anything which makes us weak, bound and narrow is unspiritual.

It is with the above goal and considerations in mind that the various rules, disciplines and standards of conduct have been formulated by many yoga teachers for their students who are of varied nature and attainments. There cannot be anything dogmatic or thoughtless about them. The goal is not to follow rules but to go beyond them. For the man of spiritual experience, ethical conduct of love, truthfulness, honesty, charity, forgiveness, trust, fearlessness, etc. are not matters of form or special effort against non-ethical or anti-social impulses. Reason, of course, plays its part, but the impetus comes not from a dry, calculating intellectualism, but from the abundant fund of selfless feeling, compassion and understanding that fills his heart.

Yoga practices are devised for purifying the mind. Purity of mind is its calmness, its freedom from restlessness and dullness. Dull and restless minds cannot attain clarity of vision. Mind is made calm and pure through acquisition of self-control by following self-imposed rules of conduct, without any other motive than purely spiritual considerations. No external rules can purify the mind unless there is a spiritual purpose behind them. The ostentatious observance of rules and forms are a sign of pride and egotism which are the opposite of spirituality. Rules do not make a yogi.

Austere practices are for attaining control of mind; they are positive in their aim like the breaking in of a vicious horse. An athlete cannot attain stamina and vigor without severe self-discipline, nor can one build the muscles of the mind without bringing it under a strict regimen.

Yoga, however, emphasizes the positive approach to mental purification. Study of scriptures is one of the great aids of mental purification. Scriptures record spiritual truths and the spiritual realizations of founders and leaders of religion. Sometimes good literature which expresses the universal truths of man and his divinity are as good as scripture. Exposing oneself to noble thoughts and association with good persons helps to bring out the higher possibilities of mind. Mind is like a piece of laundered cloth. It takes any dye easily. If it is steeped in good and positive thoughts it becomes strong and pure. Negative thoughts and materialism make it weak and cynical. For this reason daily reading of scriptures, with reflection and meditation on their passages, is among the most powerful means of self-purification.

Religious worship, prayer and recollection of the Divine Principle in us is another method of attaining calmness of mind. Austerity, study and self-dedication to the Divine are collectively called *Kriya Yoga* by the yogis. The purpose of it is to prepare the mind for samadhi by releasing it from the bonds of self-centered instincts and of egostic consciousness.

To sum up, yoga is more than ethical conduct or the observance of rules. It is actualization of the divine potentiality of man through ethical discipline and spiritual endeavor. Our moral sense gives us a glimpse of the basic solidarity of existence, the concrete realization of which is yoga. All that helps man to grow and move forward to this summit of Consciousness is part of yoga.

POSTSCRIPT ON MEDITATION

In the preceding pages I have explained the nature and purpose of meditation. Here I want to add a few more words in further comment and clarification.

Man's greatest achievement is self-mastery. People sometimes win great prizes in the world but for lack of inner peace they do not enjoy what they have gained, nor do they realize the beauty and richness of the great gift of life itself.

To feel the sweetness and greatness of life and realize the freedom we long for, we need true human development. Ambition in life is praiseworthy, but ambition that is without inner development is devoid of true meaning. After all man can realize only a few of his wishes in the world. Most people put up with their discontents and live in hopes and dreams without ever reaching and feeling what they yearn for. Poverty of spirit is a greater calamity than lack of material goods.

If we have a healthy body and a healthy mind we do not need much else to make us happy. A healthy mind is aware of the spiritual truth in us. Tagore once wrote:

My heart longs for the fulfilment of a million desires,
But ever didst Thou save me by hard refusals.
This severe grace of Thine I have stored up all my life.

Day by day Thou art making me worthy of the simple
and great gifts which Thou gavest me unasked,
This sky and the light, this body and the life and the
mind — saving me from the perils of overmuch desire.

Devil's wares are expensive,
God's gifts are without price.

Men who feel the greatness of Spirit rise above the 'discontents of civilization'; they dwell far above the petty atmosphere of little men and their little minds.

Our spiritual greatness is revealed through meditation. We often hear talk about the estrangement of the modern man from the truth of his self in the industrial and exploitative society of today where the individual has been reduced to a 'thing' or an 'object'. It is true that there has been much loss of human feeling in modern communities — apathy and lack of concern for the neighbor and the individual as such. But this is only a matter of degree. There is a deeper estrangement from Truth from which man suffers and because of which he feels fear, despair and loneliness. This estrangement is not peculiar to any society, although it may be more pronounced in one than in another.

All the great religions and spiritual philosophies speak in myths or in philosophical language of the estrangement of man from the essential truth of his nature. It is a fall from heaven; not from the heaven of nature, in whose womb man at one time lay undistinguished in primitive, preconscious existence, but from the spiritual truth of his Self. They also proclaim in myths and symbols that our freedom and salvation lie in the recovery of the original truth of our existence. Meditation is the road to our essence and freedom.

Meditation refines and deepens our feelings. Life without the capacity for feeling is vegetative existence. But uninstructed feelings and passions which are not illuminated by civilized values are also sources of pain and bondage. People therefore sometimes turn their back upon feelings — ascetics and cynics. The modern man plays safe, he does not want to get hurt. He is on the edge of life and all his talk of participation and involvement in life is a cloak that hides his rejection of it in actual deed.

Feelings need education. At the start of life we have to watch our feelings lest we be carried away helplessly on their strong and sometimes muddy tides. Meditation refines and sweetens our feelings, revealing unknown depths and beauty in them. As the bitterness of fruits changes under sun and shower into their ripened sweetness so also, under the chemistry of meditation, our raw instincts and impulses become transformed into feelings of ineffable beauty and fondness.

Man's further conquest of nature and space will bring new knowledge and comforts but it will not take him closer to his peace and happiness. Nor will it reveal the deep mystery of Being. Life will be truly wonderful and victorious if man's spiritual evolution proceeds at the same time with his material progress. Meditation is the self-conscious method of attaining the spiritual goal of life and helping the evolution of man.

V
SELECTIONS

V

SELECTIONS

THE FOLLOWING SELECTIONS have been culled from the extensive literature of yoga from the early dawn of history to our own day — a span of time stretching over five thousand years. By yoga literature I mean the writings which express the concrete and universal yogic experience of persons of profound spiritual perceptions. I have chosen a few of the highlights which were suitable for inclusion within the limits and purpose of the present book. Some of them enjoy the highest authority traditionally.

In selecting the passages I had also in mind other considerations — their beauty, their universality and their suitability for comprehension by the modern reader.

The selections may be used as objects of meditation for gaining spiritual insight and illumination.

THE VEDAS AND THE UPANISHADS

THE VEDAS, which are the earliest literature of the Indo-Aryan people, mean books of sacred knowledge and are compositions in prose and verse in archaic Sanskrit. The time of their production is uncertain but must have extended over centuries. Conservatively the vedas are assigned to a period from c. 3000 B.C. to c. 800 B.C.

The vedic literature is divided into several categories. Of these the Samhitas are the hymn portions, while the Upanishads are the final sections dealing with mystic wisdom. There are several later works bearing the name of the Upanishads and occupying themselves with philosophical topics but they are not vedic and nor do they enjoy the same authority.

In the following pages a few most significant passages from the Rigveda Samhita are given as well as the important portions of the vedic Upanishads.

THE RIGVEDA (c. 3000-2000 B.C.)

Truth is one; its expressions many.

One fire burns in many forms,
One sun lights up the whole world,
One dawn reveals all this,
One real has become all that exists.

The Hymn of Creation

Neither being nor non-being was then;
There was neither the earth, nor the interspace, nor the heavens above.
What covered all this? Where and by whom?
Was there the abyss of fathomless waters?

Death was not then, nor immortality,
Night was not yet separate from day,
Alone, that one breathed without air, self-sustained,
Beyond that nothing whatever was.

At first darkness in darkness lay hidden,
This universe was like a mass of waters undistinguished,
That which lay secret in the void became manifest through the power of his
    contemplation.

There arose first in his mind desire, the primal seed of manifestation.
The wise searching in their hearts discovered through intuition the bond
    that connects being with non-being.

Who knows and who can tell truly,
From where this universe has come and
From where it has sprung?
The gods came after creation;
Who then knows from where it came?

The source from which the universe has arisen,
Does it have a support or not?
He alone knows who is the Lord in the supreme heaven of Truth
    and self-luminous,
Maybe even He does not know!

———— . ————

We meditate the divine effulgence of the luminous Deity who pervades
    the earth, the interspace and the heavens; may the indwelling
    Spirit direct our understanding to right ends.

———— . ————

As the vision of the eye extends everywhere in space and apprehends
    all, so also do the wise see always the supreme abode of the Spirit.

The Hymn of the Goddess

This hymn is attributed to Vak, daughter of the vedic seer Ambhrina,
who experienced cosmic consciousness and spoke as follows:

I move about as the Rudras and the Vasus, the Adityas and all the other gods.
I uphold Mitra and Varuna; I am Indra, the King of the Immortals; I am Fire
    and I am the twin gods Aswins.

I am the support of the deity Soma, the destroyer of demons;
I uphold Pushan and Bhaga;
It is I who bring wealth and gifts to those who sacrifice to the gods.
I am the Ruler of all,
I bring blessings to men,
I am the Knower of Brahman,
I am the Chief among the adorables.
I exist as the manifold universe,

I am the indwelling spirit in all creatures,
I am worshipped by gods and men everywhere in different forms.
All eat and live, see and breathe and hear by My power.
Those who do not recognize Me as their indwelling spirit, they sink low in
    life.
O illustrious friend! Listen to Me
I declare to you the Truth of Brahman, attainable through faith alone.

It is I who teach the Truth of Brahman sought by gods and men.
I am the Truth;
I make him the greatest of all whom I choose.
Him I make a god, a seer, and him I fill with wisdom.

I string the bow of Rudra for the destruction of the demon Tripura, the foe
    of the good.
I battle for the sake of my worshippers.
I have entered heaven and earth as their indwelling spirit.

I have projected the heavens above.
The self-aware spirit dwelling in intelligence is my support.
Having entered all the worlds and all the beings I exist in many forms.
I pervade the far away heavens with my presence.

Having projected all this universe
I move and flow through and around it all like the wind.
Though I transcend heaven and earth yet I have become all this by My power.

KATHA UPANISHAD

Dialogue With Death

THE MOST POETICAL of the Upanishads, it gives its teachings in the setting of an ancient story. The language is clear and eloquent. It is suggested that those who are unfamiliar with this literature begin with the Katha Upanishad.

A brahmin named Vajasravasa, who followed the formal and ritualistic religion had undertaken to perform a sacrifice in which he was to give everything away. But having a stingy nature, he gave only the cows which were dry and old as presents to the priests. Noticing his father's hypocrisy, Nachiketas, a boy in his teens, enquired to whom he was to be offered, since it had been demanded that all his father's possessions be given. The father remained silent at first, but under the son's persistence finally shouted in anger, "I give you to Yama, the King of Death."

Nachiketas went dutifully to Yama's abode only to find that the King of Death was not at home. Patiently, he waited three days and nights without food. Upon his return, Yama was so distressed to find his young guest neglected that he offered to recompense Nachiketas with any three gifts the boy chose to ask.

Nachiketas demanded first that he might return to his father alive and be accepted there without anger. Second, he wished to know about a special sacrifice. And third, he asked to have the secrets of death and immortality revealed to him.

Yama was at first reluctant to disclose the ultimate secret of existence to the boy and tested him in a way which reminds one of the temptations of the Buddha and Christ. But finding that the young brahmin was a competent inquirer who had examined life and its values, Yama relented and taught Nachiketas the secret of Self.

The Upanishad belongs to about 1000 B.C. at least.

Nachiketas: There is this doubt among men about the departed; some say that he exists and others that he does not. This I would like to know under your instruction. This is the third among the boons I seek.

Yama: Even the gods had doubts about this in ancient times. This secret is too subtle to be fully grasped. Ask for another boon, Nachiketas. Do not press me. Release me from this.

Nachiketas: You say, O Death, that even the gods of old had doubts about this and that it is not easy to understand. But I will never find another teacher of this like you. No other boon can be comparable to it.

Yama: Ask for sons and grandsons who will live a hundred years; cattle, horses, elephants and gold in plenty. Ask for vast stretches of land and as long a life for yourself as you wish for.

And if you think this is a proper boon, ask for wealth and long life. O Nachiketas, prosper on this vast earth; I will fulfill all your desires.

Ask for all the objects of enjoyment which are rare in this mortal world, just as you wish — these pretty maidens with chariots and instruments of music, the like of whom men can never obtain. Be entertained by these gifts of mine but, O Nachiketas, do not ask about death.

Nachiketas: These all live for a day, O Death, and they deplete the vigor of all the senses of men. Further, life is short, however full it is. The chariots, the song and dance — let all these be yours.

Man cannot be contented by wealth. Shall we go for wealth when we have seen you? Shall we choose to live as long as you hold your sway over us? That still is the boon which I ask of you.

Having come close to imperishable eternal life, what perishable mortal here on earth below, who has seen through the pleasures of beauty and love, will take delight in a life however long it might be?

Tell us that, O Death, about which they doubt here, namely, the great passing-on. Nachiketas seeks no other boon than this which goes deep into the heart of the mystery.

Yama: The good is one and the pleasant another, both of them draw man to different ends. Of these, he who pursues the good fares well, but he who chooses the pleasant misses the goal.

Both the good and the pleasant approach a person. The wise examines and discriminates between them. The wise chooses the good over the pleasant, the simple-minded, being acquisitive and possessive, prefers the pleasant.

But you, O Nachiketas, have rejected the pleasures that are alluring after having examined them. You have not loved wealth which holds many men in the bondage of its chains.

Far apart and leading to different ends are these, ignorance and wisdom. I believe O Nachiketas, you are eager for wisdom, for even the many desires did not tempt you.

Dwelling in the midst of ignorance, wise and learned in their own esteem, the fools wander about aimlessly like the blind led by the blind.

The beyond does not manifest itself to the puerile and the stupid, deluded by the glamor of wealth. This world exists, there is no hereafter, so thinking they come under my rule over and over again.

He, of whom many do not hear even, and whom many do not understand even after hearing — wondrous is he who speaks of him and skillful is he who finds him, wondrous also is he who understands him taught by one who is skillful.

Taught by an inferior person he cannot be truly understood, being conceived in many ways. Unless taught by one who knows him as his Self, he cannot be attained, for he is beyond all conception, being subtler than the subtle.

Not by reasoning is this comprehension attainable, but dearest, taught by one who knows, it is easily understood. But you have attained it holding fast to truth. May we, O Nachiketas, find an inquirer like you!

Realizing, through the yoga of self-contemplation, the primal Divine, occult, difficult to be seen and deeply hidden in the profound depths of the heart, the wise man shakes off both pain and pleasure.

Hearing it, comprehending it and realizing the subtle truth through meditation a mortal rejoices having attained the source of joy. I believe the abode (of Self) is open to Nachiketas.

The Self, the knower, is never born, nor does he ever die. He springs from nothing; nothing springs from him. He is unborn, everlasting, eternal and primeval. He is not slain when the body is slain.

Smaller than the small, greater than the great, the Self is hidden away in the heart of a creature. The person who is without desire sees the Self and his greatness, freed from sorrow and through tranquility of mind.

This Self cannot be attained by instruction, nor by intellectual power, nor by much learning. He is attained by him whom the Self chooses. To such a one, the Self reveals his own nature.

He who has not ceased from evil doing, he who is not tranquil, he who is not meditative, and he whose mind is not peaceful, can never attain the Self through intuition.

Know the Self as the rider in the chariot and the body as the chariot, know the intellect as the charioteer and the mind as the reins.

The senses are called the horses, the sense-objects their paths; the Self in conjunction with the body, the senses, and the mind is said to be the experiencer (the empirical person) by the wise.

He who has no understanding and whose mind is never calm, his senses are out of control like the wicked horses of a charioteer.

But he who has understanding and whose mind is ever tranquil, his senses are under control like the good horses of a charioteer.

He who has no understanding, whose mind is scattered and who is always impure, he does not attain the goal but wanders through rounds of existence.

But he who has understanding, whose mind is collected and who is ever pure, he attains that goal from which there is no more any descent into empirical existence.

The man whose intellect, the charioteer, holds the reins of mind in a firm grasp, he reaches the journey's end, the supreme abode of the all-prevading spirit.

Beyond the senses are the sense-objects; beyond the objects is the mind; beyond the mind is the intellect; beyond the intellect is the cosmic Self.

Beyond the great (cosmic) Self is the unmanifest; beyond the unmanifest is the spirit. Beyond the spirit there is nothing. That is the limit; that is the final goal. (See the chapter on *Nature*).

The Self, hidden in all beings, is not manifest, but is seen by persons of subtle perception through their supreme and subtle intelligence.

The wise should merge speech in mind, the latter in the intellect, the intellect in the cosmic Self; the cosmic Self he should merge in the tranquil Self.

Arise, awake and having approached the best of teachers comprehend it. Sharp as the razor's edge and difficult to cross, the sages declare that it is a hard road to travel.

The Self-existent Spirit made the senses outgoing; therefore one looks outward and does not see the Self within. But some rare sage, seeking life eternal, saw the inner Self with introverted vision.

The simple-minded run after outward pleasures and walk into the widespread snare of death. But the wise, knowing immortal life, do not seek here the eternal among things which are fleeting.

Whatever is here is also there, whatever is there is also here. He goes from death to death, who perceives the one as many here.

By mind alone is this to be attained. There is no multiplicity here at all. He who perceives manyness here goes from death to death.

As fire which is one becomes varied, upon entering the world, according to the fuel it consumes, so also the inner Self of all beings though one, becomes many according to the form it enters and pervades.

Just as the sun which is the eye of the whole world is not tainted by the faults the eye sees outside, so also the one inner Self of all is not touched by the outer pain of the world.

The one, the Ruler, the inner Self of all, who makes the one seed manifold — the wise who see Him as abiding in their Self, to them belongs eternal bliss and to none other.

The one eternal amid the transient, the Conscious amid the many conscious, the One among the many, the Providence — the wise who perceive Him in their Self, to them belongs eternal peace and to none other.

The sun does not shine there, nor the moon and the stars, nor do lightnings flash there, what to speak of this fire? He shining, everything shines. All this becomes manifest by His light.

This sempiternal asvattha (peepul) tree has its roots above and branches below. That is the Pure, that is Brahman. And that indeed is called Immortal. In it rest all the worlds; nothing transcends it. This indeed is that.

All that lives and moves in the world (the world process) has sprung from Prana (life, the cosmic energy). It is the great fear like the upraised thunderbolt (the world process moves as it were under fear; i.e. is governed by Prana). They who know this become immortal.

His form does not dwell in the field of vision; no one ever sees Him with the eye. Framed by feeling, thought and intelligence, those who know Him become immortal. (The Divine which is beyond all conception is formed by different natures according to their feeling and intelligence).

When the five senses of knowledge and the mind cease from functioning, and even the intellect does not act — that, they say, is the highest state.

This they regard as yoga — the steady control of the senses. Then one has perfect Awareness, for yoga (concentration) comes and goes.

Not by speech, not by mind, nor by the eye can He be apprehended. How can He be comprehended except as Existence (except in the fashion of one who says "He is").

He should be apprehended as Pure Existence alone and in His own true nature. His true nature becomes clear to one who apprehends Him as pure Existence.

When all the desires which dwell in his heart depart, then the mortal becomes immortal and even here he unites with the Brahman.

When all the knots of the heart are sundered here, then the mortal becomes immortal. This is the ultimate teaching.

ISHA UPANISHAD (c. 1000 B.C.)

ONE OF THE SMALLEST of the Upanishads, it has had a profound influence upon Indian life. The great leaders of modern India like Tagore and Gandhi drew inspiration from it.

It proclaims the essential unity of God and the world, spirit and nature, and sanctifies life and activity by teaching that the Divine dwells everywhere.

INVOCATION

The Beyond is infinite; manifestation is infinite. The infinite emanates from the infinite. Taking the infinite from the infinite the infinite remains.

All this, whatever there is in this changing universe (Jagat or process), is pervaded by the Divine. Therefore, find enjoyment through renunciation (of egoistic self-will); do not covet another's possession.

Doing work here on earth a man should wish to live a hundred years. There is no other way for you except this by which you will not be bound by work.

Sunless and hidden in blind gloom are the worlds where those who deny the Spirit go after death.

The Spirit is one, immobile and swifter than the mind. The senses never reach it, which is ever ahead of them. Standing still it outstrips all others though they move fast. Because of it, the world-spirit upholds the actions of all beings.

It moves and yet does not move; it is far and yet it is near. It is within all this and it is also outside all this.

But he who sees all beings in the Self and the Self in all things, he does not thereafter hate anyone.

When all beings have become one with his Self, how can he, the knower, who sees only unity, have any delusion or sorrow?

KENA UPANISHAD (c. 1000 B.C.)

IN THIS UPANISHAD the teacher instructs the disciple on the subtle nature of Brahman which is the one Self of all and the one Power behind all powers.

He who is the ear of the ear, the mind of the mind, the speech of speech, He is also the life of life and the eye of the eye. The wise, therefore, giving up self-identification with the senses, attain eternal life after death.

There the eye does not go, nor speech, nor even the mind. He is not the object of our knowledge, nor can we teach Him to others. He is other than the known; other than the unknown also. So have we heard from former teachers who explained it to us. (The Spirit is pure subject and can never be known as an object.)

That which is not expressed by speech but which manifests speech (the silence which makes communication possible), know that to be Brahman and not what people adore here.

That which is not thought of by the mind, but which manifests the mind, know that to be Brahman and not what people adore here.

That which the eye does not see but because of which the eye sees, know that to be Brahman and not what people adore here.

That which the ear does not hear but because of which the ear hears, know that to be Brahman and not what people adore here.

That which is not supported by life but by which life is supported, know that to be Brahman and not what people adore here.

If you think that you have known Brahman well, you know it but little for you have known only its manifested and limited forms. So it is still to be examined and reflected upon, so I (the teacher) think.

Disciple: I do not think that I have known Brahman well, nor that I do not know it at all. He who among us understands the sense of the expression, "It is neither that I know, nor that I do not know," he alone understands Brahman.

Whosoever thinks that he does not know Brahman, he understands it and he who thinks he knows it, he does not understand it. It is not understood by those who know but is understood by them who do not know.

When it is known in every state of awareness (as the silent witness) then it is truly known, through such knowledge one attains eternal life. Through one's Self one gains power; through wisdom one gains immortality.

If a man knows Brahman here on earth then he finds the Truth, but if he does not know he comes to great grief. Perceiving the Real in all the beings, the wise attain eternal life departing from this world.

The following is an illustration of the knowledge of Brahman. The manifestation and realization of Brahman is (sudden) like a flash of lightning or the winking of an eye...

Austerities, self-control and work are its (the Upanishad's, i.e., of self-knowledge) support, the vedas (scriptures) are its limbs and Truth is its abode.

THE MUNDAKA UPANISHAD (c. 1000 B.C.)

THIS UPANISHAD after drawing a clear distinction between the higher knowledge of Spirit and the lower knowledge of nature, the world process, points out the nature of Self, the means of achieving self-knowledge and its result.

...Two kinds of knowledge are to be known, so the knowers of Brahman (Spirit) declare — the higher as well as the lower (the noumenal and the phenomenal).

This is the Truth. As thousands of sparks of similar form emanate from a blazing fire, so also, O beloved, beings of different kinds arise from the imperishable and into that they depart again.

The Divine Person is formless; He is within and without and unborn. He is beyond life, beyond mind, luminous and supreme, beyond the immutable (unmanifested nature).

From Him are born life, mind, and the senses, ether, air, fire, water and earth, the supporter of all.

Manifest and dwelling secretly in the hearts of all is the Supreme Spirit. All that moves, breathes and winks rest in It. Know this as being and as non-being, as the supremely desirable and as the highest wisdom above the science of man.

That which is luminous, that which is subtler than the subtle, that in which the worlds and the dwellers in them rest, that is the imperishable Brahman. That is life; that is speech and mind. That is Truth; that is immortal and that is to be known, O beloved. Realize that.

Taking as the bow the mighty weapon of the Upanishads, the arrow sharpened by meditation, and drawing it with a mind absorbed in contemplation of It (the Spirit), aim, O beloved, at the imperishable Brahman as the target.

Aum (or Om, the sacred syllable, the sound symbol of Brahman) is the bow, the soul (individual) is the arrow, and the Brahman is its target. One should pierce it with an unfaltering aim and become one with it like the arrow which has penetrated its target.

He in whom the heavens, the earth and the interspace are woven along with the mind and all the life forces, realize him alone, the one Self, give up other talks. This is the bridge to immortality.

Where the channels of life's currents (nerves and arteries) join together like the spokes in the nave of a chariot-wheel, there he, the Self, dwells within, manifesting himself in diverse ways. Meditate on Aum as the Self. May success be yours in crossing over to the shore beyond darkness. (The Self is to be meditated upon at the heart center. See the chapter on meditation).

Framed by the mind, the leader of life and body, He dwells in matter (the body) controlling the heart. The wise through self-knowledge see clearly the Blissful, the Immortal and the Luminous Spirit.

When one sees the Transcendent Spirit, the knot of his heart is sundered, all his doubts are dispelled and his acts (egoistic deeds) terminate.

Two birds of beautiful plumage, friends and inseparable companions, dwell on the self-same tree. Of these two, one eats the sweet fruits, the other looks on without eating.

On the self-same tree, a person grieves, immersed helplessly in the sorrows of the world from delusion. But when he sees the other, the beloved, the Lord and His greatness, his sorrows pass away.

When the seer perceives the Lord of golden color, the Person and the source of Brahma (world-soul, the first born), then he, the knower, leaving behind good and evil, becomes taintless and attains the supreme identity.

He is Life of life (prana) who shines through all beings. Knowing him the wise man recoils from words; sporting in the Self, delighting in the Self and active, he is the best among the knowers of Brahman. (The wise man who is active is superior to all).

The Self, luminous and pure and dwelling in the body, is attainable by truth, self-discipline, integral knowledge and purity. He is seen by the yogis whose impurities have melted away.

Truth alone triumphs, falsehood never. By truth has been laid out the way to the Divine—the road along which the sages, whose desires have been fulfilled, travel to where lies the supreme abode of Truth.

The Spirit is vast and divine and unthinkable. Subtler than the subtle it is manifest in many ways. It is farther than the far, yet is here close to us; for those who have vision it dwells in the secret depths of the heart.

The Self is not grasped by the eye, nor even by speech, nor by other sense-organs, nor by austerity, nor by work. But when one's inner being is purified by the serenity of wisdom then alone does he see the formless spirit through contemplation.

This subtle Self is to be known by the pure mind in the body where the life force has entered and has become diversified into the five sense-functions. Sense-functions pervade the mind (psyche) of all beings. When the mind is purified, the Self becomes manifest.

He who seeks enjoyments, his mind dwelling on desires, is born wherever they drag him. But of the man whose desires have been fulfilled and who has found the Self, all his longings vanish even here on earth.

This Self cannot be attained by instruction, nor by intellectual power, nor by much learning of scripture (theological learning). He is attained by one whom the Self chooses. To him the Self reveals its nature.

This Self cannot be attained by the weak, nor through heedlessness nor by thoughtless asceticism. But the man of understanding who strives by these means, this Self of his enters into Brahman, its abode.

Having attained Him, the seers, happy with their knowledge and self-fulfilled, are without passion and tranquil. These wise and self-established yogis unite with all after having found the all-pervading spirit everywhere.

Just as the flowing rivers enter into the ocean losing their name and form so also the wise, free from name and form (limitations of nature), attain the Supreme Divine Person.

CHHANDOGYA UPANISHAD (c. 1200 B.C.)

THE VAST PORTION OF this Upanishad is occupied with various forms of vedic *upasana* or method of worship and meditation on the different symbols of Spirit, which are rather archaic and relative to a cultural milieu, local and of the past, and therefore have little universal significance.

There are however, several passages dealing with the knowledge of Brahman from which the following are taken.

IN THE OLDEN DAYS there was a young person called Shvetaketu, the son of Aruni. His father said to him: "Shvetaketu, live the life of a religious student. No one in our family, dear one, is without learning and a Brahmin by birth alone."

Shvetaketu became a pupil at the age of twelve, and having studied all the vedas returned home when he was twenty-four, greatly conceited, arrogant and thinking himself learned.

His father said to him, "Shvetaketu, I see you are conceited and arrogant and think yourself well-read. But did you seek that instruction by which that which cannot be thought of becomes thought of and that which cannot be known becomes known?"

Shvetaketu replied, "What kind of instruction is that?"

"Just as, my dear, by one clod of clay all that is made of clay becomes known, the modification being only nominal, a matter of speech, while the truth is that it is only clay.

"Just as, my dear, by a nugget of gold all that is made of gold becomes known, the modification being only nominal, a matter of speech, while the truth is that it is only gold.

"Just as, my dear, by a pair of nail clippers all that is made of iron becomes known, the modification being only nominal, a matter of speech, while the truth is that it is only iron; such, O dear, is the instruction."

Shvetaketu: "Truly the revered teachers did not know this, for if they had known it why would not they have told it to me. Please, sir, tell that to me."

"Let it be so," said he.

"In the beginning, my dear, before creation there was Being alone, one without a second. About this some others say, "In the beginning before creation there was non-being alone, one without a second, from that Being was born."

"But how indeed, my dear, can this be?" said he. "How from non-being could Being arise?" Truly, my dear, there was Being alone, one without a second, before creation."

"The whole world has as its soul, that subtle essence. That is the Truth, that is the Self. You are that, O Shvetaketu."

Aruni: "Bring a fruit from that banyan tree."

Shvetaketu: "Here it is, sir."

Aruni: "Break it."

Shvetaketu: "It is broken, sir."

Aruni: "Break one of them (the seed) my child."

Shvetaketu: "It is broken, sir."

Aruni: "What do you see there?"

Shvetaketu: "Nothing at all, sir."

Aruni said to him, "My dear, the subtle essence of the seed which you do not see, from that subtle essence this banyan tree has arisen. Believe me, my dear."

"These eastern rivers, my dear, flow toward the east and the western toward west. They rise from the ocean and into the ocean they go. They become the ocean. Just as the rivers merged in the ocean do not know, "I am this river, I am that river," so also, my dear, all these creatures arising from Being do not know, "We have arisen from Being." "The whole world has for its self that subtle essence. That is the Truth. That is the Self. You are that, O Shvetaketu."

Aruni: Place this salt in water and come to me in the morning. Shvetaketu did that. The father said, Son, bring the salt which you placed in the water last evening.

He could not find it even after searching, though it was there dissolved in water.

Father: Take a sip from the top; how is it?

Son: Salty.

Father: Take a sip from the middle; how is it? Son: Salty.

Father: Take a sip from the bottom, how is it? Son: Salty.

Father: Throw it away and sit near me. He did so saying, "The salt was there always."

Father said to him, "Just as you could not find the salt though it is in the water so also, my dear, the Pure Being is here in this body—here indeed."

*   *   *

Narada approached Sanatkumara and said, "Venerable sir, please instruct me."

Sanatkumara said to him, "Tell me what you have learned. I will instruct you what is beyond."

Narada said: Sir, I know the Rigveda, Yajurveda, Samaveda, Atharvaveda, the fourth (veda), epic and ancient lore, the fifth, grammar, ancestral rites, arithmetic, science of omens, chronology (science of time), logic, ethics and politics, theology, vedic scholarship, science of elements, the science of weapons, astronomy, science of serpents and fine arts. All this I know, sir.

But sir, I am, with all this learning, like one who knows only the words but not the Self. I have heard from wise men like you that the knower of Self crosses over sorrow. Sir, I am one who is sorrowful. Please help me to cross over sorrow.

Sanatkumara told him: Whatever you have learned is only a name (i.e. it is only phenomenal knowledge and not the knowledge of Substance or Reality).

Narada: Is there, sir, anything higher than name?

Sanatkumara: There is something higher than name.

Narada: Tell me that, sir.

Sanatkumara: That which is infinite is happiness. There is no happiness in the finite. The infinite alone is happiness. One should, therefore, desire to know the infinite.

Where one sees nothing else, hears nothing else, knows nothing else, that is the infinite. But where one sees something else, hears something else, knows something else, that is the finite. That which is infinite is immortal; that which is finite is mortal.

Narada: Sir, where is the infinite established?

Sanatkumara: It is established in its own majesty or not even there.

The infinite is below; it is above; it is behind; it is in front; it is to the south, it is the north—it is indeed all this (world).

I am below; I am above; I am behind; I am in front; I am to the south; I am to the north; I am all this (the Self is infinite).

Now here, in this body, the city of Brahman, is a tiny abode, the lotus of the heart. Within it is the tiny inner space of Brahman. One should seek that which is within the lotus of the heart. That indeed is what one should desire to know well.

If they (the disciples) should say to him (the teacher): "What is it which dwells in the small inner space within the lotus of the heart in the city of Brahman that we should seek and desire to understand?" Then he should reply: "The space within the heart extends as much as this space of the universe extends. Heaven and earth, fire and air, sun and moon, lightning and stars are all within it. Whatever of him is here and whatever not, all that is contained in it."

BRIHAD ARANYAKA UPANISHAD (c. 1200 B.C.)

IT IS THE LARGEST of the Upanishads and traditionally the most important. Its three sections deal with the basic identity of the individual with the universal spirit, philosophical justification of this view and methods of worship and meditation.

> ...Lead me from the unreal to the real,
> ...Lead me from darkness to light,
> ...Lead me from death to immortality...

At that time (i.e., before creation), this universe was unmanifest. It became differentiated through name and form. Even now the differentiation is formal and linguistic as it is said, "This is his name" and "This is his shape." He has entered into this universe even up to the tip of its nails just as a razor is hidden in the razor case and fire in the fuel. People do not see Him because what they see is limited. When breathing He is called life; when speaking, voice; when seeing, the eye; when hearing, the ear; when thinking, the mind. These are merely the names of His acts. He who meditates, meditates on one or another of these aspects he does not know, for the Self is incomplete when qualified by one or other of these attributes. Therefore meditate on Him as the Self for in Him all these unite. This Self is to be known. It is the goal of all beings, for by knowing it, one knows all.

It is because of the Self that all is dear to us. The Self, O Maitreyi, should be seen, should be heard of, reflected on and meditated upon. Dear one, when the Self is seen through hearing, reflection and contemplation, all this is known.

Where there is duality as it were (in the time of manifestation), there one smells another, one sees another, one hears another, one speaks to another, one thinks of another and one knows another. But when all has become his Self then by what and whom will one smell, by what and whom will one see, by what and whom will one hear, by what and whom will one speak, by what and whom will one think, by what and whom will one know? By what can one know that by which all this is known? By what, my dear, can the knower be known?

This very Self is the overlord of all beings, the King of them all. Just as all the spokes of a chariot wheel are held together in its nave and rim, so also all the creatures, all the gods, all the worlds, all the senses and all the individual selves are held together by the supreme Self.

As one acts and behaves so does one become. He who does good becomes good; he who does evil becomes evil. One becomes virtuous by virtuous actions, evil by evil actions. Men of discernment also say: "An individual is made up of desires. As is his desire, so is his will; as is his will so is his act, and as he acts so does he reap."

When all the desires which dwell in his heart are cast away then a mortal becomes immortal and attains Brahman even here in this body.

It is to be perceived by the mind alone. There is no manifoldness in it at all. He who sees manifoldness in it goes from death to death.

Eternal and beyond rational demonstration, it is to be perceived as one alone. The great Self is without stain, higher than the unmanifest, unborn and eternal.

This great Self is without birth and without decay; it is the immortal, eternal, and fearless Brahman. The Brahman is fearless. He who knows this becomes the fearless Brahman.

SHVETASHVATARA UPANISHAD (c. 800 B.C.)

THIS UPANISHAD PROCLAIMS the unity of existence, of the world and the many beings, in the one Supreme Spirit. It emphasizes the personal aspect of the Godhead for purposes of worship. The Divine is the *mayin,* the lord of maya, the maker who makes the world. Nature is God's power. Many yoga concepts, later clearly formulated and now current, are first found here. It is a most poetical composition as well.

The philosophers of Brahman inquire: Is Brahman the cause (of the world)? From where do we come? By what do we live? And where de we finally rest? Under whose dispensation and governed by whom do we experience pain and pleasure?

Time, nature, necessity, chance, the elements and the individual soul — are they the cause? A conjunction of these cannot be the cause, because the soul is the cause of conjunction (soul is the organizing principle of life). Nor is soul the cause because it is powerless and subject to pleasure and pain. (The unconscious cannot be the cause of the conscious, the unintelligent of the intelligent, nor does the individual determine his own destiny).

Failing to discover the first cause through reason, thè enquirers of Brahman saw through the yoga of contemplation the self-power of the Deity constituted of the three gunas — the Deity who governs and regulates all the factors mentioned before, from time to the soul.

Thinking that it is different from the Prime Mover, the individual self wanders and revolves in the great wheel of Brahman, the origin and the end of all living beings. But the same soul, knowing itself as one with the Deity, gains life eternal.

The Lord upholds this universe of perishable and imperishable, manifest and unmanifest states, which are related, one to the other, as cause and effect. Under the delusion of ignorance the individual soul becomes bound by the egoistic sense of being both doer and enjoyer. But by knowing the Divine he is freed from all fetters.

The Supreme Spirit has assumed the forms of the omniscient Lord as well as the individual self of the ignorant, which are both eternal. There is another eternal principle, Nature (the power of Brahman), which provides the field of experience to the soul. The Supreme Spirit is infinite, of cosmic form and above action. When the individual knows the three — the individual, the Lord and Nature as the Brahman — he is freed from all fetters.

Nature is perishable, the Lord is imperishable. The One Divinity governs both the perishable nature and the imperishable soul. From repeated contemplation of Him, from joining with Him and from knowing Him as one's Self, one becomes free from the illusory knowledge of the world.

Regarding these three, the empirical self, the objects of experience, and the Prime Mover as Brahman, as proclaimed by the teachers, know the Divine as dwelling always in the Self. There is nothing beyond this to be known.

As the form of fire latent in the wood is not seen and yet its potency is not lost, because it can be manifested again through friction, so also the Supreme Spirit can be realized in this body by means of Aum (Om).

Holding the head, the neck and the chest erect and the body even and withdrawing the senses and the mind into the heart, the wise should cross the dreadful torrents of the world in the raft of Brahman (Aum).

During the practice of yoga forms of fog, smoke, sun, air, fire, fireflies, lightning, crystal, the moon and the like come as the indications of Brahman.

When the subtle truth of the elements becomes manifest to the yogi, he attains a body purified by the fire of yoga; for him there is no more disease, decrepitude or death.

When the contemplative yogi perceives in his heart the luminous Brahman as his own Self, then knowing the Divine who is birthless and changeless and devoid of all attributes, he is freed from all fetters.

This all-pervasive Divinity becomes the first-born, the world-soul; He also becomes the cosmos. He has been born and will be born again as the young ones. And as the indwelling Spirit of all, he has his face turned in every direction.

The Deity who is in fire and who is in water, and who has entered into the entire universe; He who is in annuals and who is in perennials — Him we salute again and again.

The One who holds all the worlds in His magic net and governs them by his lordly powers, who remains the same while worlds arise and perish — they who know this become immortal.

He who is the source and support of the gods, who is the Lord of cosmos, who is Rudra, the great seer, and who of old produced the world-soul, may He endow us with right understanding.

I have known the Supreme Person of sunlike splendor beyond darkness. Only by knowing Him does one cross over death. There is no other way of reaching there.

Than whom there is nothing higher, than whom there is nothing subtler; He who stands still like a tree established in His own self-luminous glory — by Him is this whole universe pervaded.

That which is far beyond the world is without form and without trouble. Those who know that gain eternal life; others who do not, come only to grief.

The inner self of all is of the measure of a thumb, ever dwelling in the hearts of men, framed by thought and feeling. Those who know this become immortal.

The Person is all this, all that has been, all that will be and all that is now. He is also the Lord of immortality.

Reflecting the qualities of the senses, yet devoid of them all, He is the Lord and Ruler and the great support of all.

Without feet and hands He moves fast and grasps all. He sees without eye, hears without ear. He knows all that is knowable, but no one knows Him. The knowers of Brahman call Him the Primeval, the Supreme Person.

Subtler than the subtle, greater than the great the Self is hidden away in the heart of all beings. When a person beholds the tranquil Lord and His majesty through purity of heart, he becomes free from sorrow.

I know the undecaying, ancient Self of all dwelling everywhere by His all-pervasive presence whom the knowers of Brahman proclaim to be birthless and eternal.

He who is one and without form but who sportingly creates the manifold universe by his myriad powers, He in whom the universe exists and to whom it departs at the end is the Divine Person. May He endow us with the right understanding.

You are the woman, you are the man; you are the youth, you are the maiden too. You are the old man tottering on a staff. Being born you assume diverse forms.

You are the dark bluebird, you are the red-eyed green parrot. You are the thunderladen cloud, You are the seasons and You are the oceans. You are without beginning; Your presence pervades everything. It is from You that all the worlds have come into being.

Know Nature to be maya, the Power of God, and the Supreme Lord, the Master of maya. This entire universe is pervaded by beings who form parts of Him.

He indeed is the Protector of the world in time, the Ruler of all, secretly hidden in all beings, in whom are united the seers and the gods. Knowing Him one sunders the bonds of death.

This God, the world-maker, the great Self, dwells always in the hearts of all. He becomes manifest through instruction, through discrimination and through reflection. Those who know Him become immortal.

When there is no darkness (ignorance), there is neither day nor night, neither being nor non-being; He, the Pure and changeless, is then alone. That is the imperishable and adorable light; and from Him has flowed the perennial wisdom into the hearts of the wise.

His form does not dwell in the ken of vision, no one ever sees Him with the eye. Those who know Him thus, as seated in the heart, through pure feeling and reason, they become immortal.

As the sun shines resplendent illuminating the regions above and below and across, so also the Divine Lord, one and adorable, governs all that originates from His powers.

The truth of Self is hidden in the Upanishads, the secret section of the vedas. The world-soul knows it, the source of wisdom. Those gods and seers of yore who knew it became immortal by uniting with it.

The individual self is to be conceived as a part of the hundreth part of the point of a hair divided a hundredfold. Yet it is infinite in its true nature.

It is not a woman, nor a man, nor a neuter. Whatever body it takes to itself, it is identified with it.

Coming to know the Divine, who is without beginning and end, who dwells in the whirl of the world, who is the creator of the universe, who assumes diverse forms and who pervades all, one is freed from all fetters.

Some thinkers say that Nature is the cause (of all); others who are deluded say it is Time. But it is the majesty of the Lord in the world which turns the wheel of the universe.

The Lord has neither body nor sense organs. There is none equal or superior to Him. His divine power (maya) of creative consciousness is manifold and inherent in His nature.

There is no master, nor ruler of Him in the world. Nor is there a sign by which he can be known. He is the Prime cause, the Lord of the individual self. He has no progenitor, nor has He any overlord.

May the one God who has covered Himself with various names and forms by His own power like a spider covers itself with its threads, may He unite us with Brahman.

The one God is hidden in all beings. He is all-pervasive, the inner self of all, the ordainer of deeds, the final abode of all beings, the witness of all, the light of consciousness, the only one and devoid of attributes.

He who is the one controller of the many who are without self-movement, He who makes manifest the one seed — the wise who see Him abiding in their own self, to them belongs eternal happiness, and to none else.

He is the Eternal among eternals (individual selves), the Intelligent among the intelligences, the One among many, who grants desires. Knowing the Prime Cause, the Divine, attainable through discrimination and contemplation (samkhya and yoga), one is freed from all fetters.

The sun does not shine there, nor the moon, nor the stars. These lightnings do not flash there, what to speak of this fire? Because He shines, everything shines after Him; by His light all this is lighted.

There is only one Self in this universe. He is the fire dwelling within the waters (body). Knowing Him one crosses over death, there is no other way to reach there.

He is the world-maker, the knower of all, the self-caused, the light of Consciousness, the maker of time, the Good, the all-knower, the lord of nature and soul, the master of the gunas (forces of nature) and the cause of liberation from worldly existence as well as of the bondage of the world.

When men shall roll up the sky like a piece of leather then alone they shall come to the end of their sorrow without knowing the Divine. He is the highest bridge to immortality; who is without parts, without action, tranquil and flawless and without blemish like a fire which has devoured its fuel.

By the power of austerity and by the grace of God, the sage Shetashvatara realized the supreme and pure Brahman and spoke of it fully to the ascetics — the truth that is dear to all the seers.

The highest mystery of the Upanishads which was declared in a former cycle, should not be imparted to one who is not calm nor to one who is not a son or a disciple.

He who has the supreme devotion to the Deity and the same to the teacher as to the Deity, to that great soul the truths spoken in the Upanishads become manifest — to him do they become manifest.

THE GITA

THE GITA is the most popular scripture of the Hindus. It is a book of seven hundred verses and is in the form of a dialogue between the teacher Krishna and the disciple Arjuna. Both teacher and disciple were princes from the warrior class of Kshatriyas.

The Gita is a small part of the much larger Hindu Epic, THE MAHABHARATA, which contains 100,000 verses in its present recension. The epic was written round a great battle which was fought between two sets of royal cousins and their followers over a disputed kingdom in northern India about 1500 B.C.

The Gita literally means a song. It is often respectfully called the Bhagavad Gita or the Song of the Lord, i.e., the divine teachings of Sri Krishna. According to tradition, Sri Krishna delivered his teachings to Arjuna on the field of battle. Therefore, a modern writer has called it "The Sermon on the Battlefield."

THE MAHABHARATA contains many other smaller gitas or poetical compositions. They are spiritual teachings attributed to persons of wisdom and illumination, men and women. Sri Krishna delivered another sermon, the Anu Gita, which is shorter and not so famous but also contained in the same epic.

The occasion of the Gita was the confrontation of Arjuna with the enemy army in battle array, which included his cousins, teachers, superiors, friends and others. It was an old Kshatriya custom to fight according to a code — to greet and salute opponents in battle before engaging in war and to strike straight from the shoulder.

Sri Krishna was Arjuna's charioteer and was with him. Arjuna became overwhelmed with emotion at the sight of his relatives on the enemy field. Though he was the chief general and head of his army, he refused to fight, maintaining that it was bad to kill one's relatives and friends, to engage in civil war and wade through a pool of blood to kingdom and fortune. He declared he would rather renounce both war and the world and become a mendicant.

It was at this point that Sri Krishna began to speak. He urged Arjuna to fight for his king and country, not from a mere sense of duty alone but from that higher spiritual attitude and vision which is the ultimate source and justification of all ethical rules.

Arjuna's question was not just a limited moral question. He was a spiritual seeker. He saw a contradiction between the spiritual ideal and the violence of war imposed upon him by his duty and position. The Gita is Krishna's answer to his perplexities.

The Gita reconciles action with contemplation. It sanctifies and hallows the world and everyday life. It affirms the uniqueness of individuality in the context of the impersonal. It gives the essence of yoga. It calls itself a yoga shastra, i.e., the scripture of yoga.

After the Bible, the Gita is the most widely translated book in the world. It has influenced many minds in many lands. When Carlyle met Emerson, he presented the latter with a copy of the Gita. In the early editions of her book, SCIENCE AND HEALTH, Mary Baker Eddy used to have quotations from the Gita. Many New England spiritual movements owe much to it.

Sri Krishna, the spokesman of the Gita, is one of the great spiritual leaders of India. He is regarded by the Hindus as an incarnation, as a special manifestation of Divinity. Sri Krishna affirms in the Gita that the Divine Power steps on the stage of human history from time to time as an incarnation for the preservation of right and the destruction of evil. The world order is preserved and creative advance takes place when vision is combined with strength (brahma kshatra). The Gita proclaims that, despite all appearances to the contrary, truth and justice are bound to prevail. Man achieves freedom by becoming a willing instrument of the Divine.

The Gita is thought to have been composed before the time of the Buddha, in the sixth century B.C. The MAHABHARATA as we have it today is not the work of a single author or age. It grew to its present size in the course of centuries through additions to an original core. The Gita belongs to the earlier period of its composition.

There are many translations of the Gita in all the western languages. The best English translations are by Sir Edwin Arnold called The Song Celestial and by Sri Sarvepalli Radhakrishnan, the present President of India (1963). Sir Edwin's translation is unexcelled from the poetical point of view, but Radhakrishnan's version is the most suitable for modern readers.

Below are given most of the verses of the Gita, chapter by chapter. The translation is mine. I have attempted to give a faithful rendering. However, I must add that there cannot be any literal translation from one language to another, especially when technical and cultural terms and notions are concerned. The color, the tone of a word or phrase and the various associations and meanings that collect round them in a particular culture due to its peculiar experience, cannot be conveyed by simple literal translation. All that can be done is to convey the exact sense as gracefully and economically as possible.

When Krishna refers to himself he means the Supreme Spirit both in its impersonal and transcendant aspect as also in the personal aspect of the Lord of Creation.

I

Chapter I is called Arjuna's lament. It portrays his distress and bewilderment at the sight of his opponents in the battlefield. Overcome with pity and confusion he refuses to fight.

II

KRISHNA:
Do not, O Arjuna, give way to unmanliness. It does not become you. Give up this petty weakness of heart and arise, O subduer of enemies!

ARJUNA:
Overcome with sentimental weakness and bewildered about the right thing to do, I ask you. Tell me for certain what is good. I am your disciple, teach me who have taken refuge in you.

SPIRIT & BODY

KRISHNA:

You are lamenting those for whom there should be no grief, and yet you speak words of wisdom. Wise men do not grieve for the dead or for the living.

There never was a time when I did not exist, nor you, nor these rulers of men. And there never will be a time hereafter when we shall all cease to be.

As the soul goes through childhood, youth, and old age in this body, so also does it pass into another. The wise man cherishes no delusions about them.

Sense contacts, O Arjuna, give rise to feelings of heat and cold, pleasure and pain. They come and go and are fleeting. Bear them lightly.

One who is not affected by these, O Chief among men, and who is wise, being the same in pain and pleasure, becomes fit for eternal life.

The unreal never comes into being; the Real never ceases to exist. The final truth of both of these has been seen by men of subtle perceptions.

Know that to be Imperishable by which all this has been pervaded. None whatsoever can annihilate this Immutable being.

The bodies of the eternal embodied Spirit which is imperishable and imponderable, are said to have an end. Therefore fight, O Arjuna.

He who knows it to be a slayer and he also who thinks it is slain — both of them do not know. It neither slays nor is slain.

It is never born, nor does it die; nor does it ever cease to be after having come to exist. Without birth, eternal, everlasting and primeval, it is never slain when the body is slain.

How can a person, O Arjuna, who knows it to be imperishable, eternal, without birth and without decay, slay one or cause another to slay.

Just as a man puts on new clothes discarding the ones worn out, so also the embodied spirit enters into other bodies that are new, relinquishing the ones worn out.

Weapons do not sunder it, fire does not burn it, water does not melt it, nor does air evaporate it.

It cannot be sundered or burnt; it cannot be melted or dried up. It is eternal and omnipresent, changeless and immovable and the same as always. It is declared to be unmanifest, incomprehensible and unchanging. Therefore knowing it to be so you should not grieve.

Some look upon it as if in wonder, others likewise speak of it in wonder, and also in wonder yet others hear of it; and even after hearing, none whatsoever comprehends it.

The indwelling spirit in the body of everyone is eternal and cannot be slain, O Arjuna. Therefore you should not grieve for any being.

And having regard to your duty also, you should not quail. There is nothing higher for a kshatriya (warrior) than a war which comes as a call of duty.

THE WISDOM OF YOGA

Treating alike pleasure and pain, gain and loss, victory and defeat, prepare yourself for battle. Thus you will not incur sin.

This is the wisdom of the samkhya which has just been spoken to you. Now listen to the wisdom of yoga. Equipped with this understanding, O Arjuna, you will cast away the bondage of work (karma).

(Samkhya and yoga are not different. But sometimes the view of reality and the method of realization are distinguished as samkya and yoga. In practice they are one.)

In the practice of yoga no effort is lost, nor is there any obstacle. Even a little of this dharma (practice) saves one from great fear.

In yoga, O Arjuna, the conviction is only one and inflexible, but the views of the irresolute are many-branched and endless.

The undiscerning ones recite the flowery words of the vedas, full of numerous, special and complicated rites for gaining enjoyment and power, and which lead to rebirth as the result of works. These men are filled with desire and intent upon heaven; they revel in the lore of the vedas and deny that there is anything else (beside, that is, the religion of heaven).

The minds of those who are attached to enjoyment and power and whose hearts have been carried away by the vedic words are not given to illumination.

The vedas deal with the world of process (the gunas). But Arjuna, go beyond the realm of gunas. Be free from all dualities and ever established in truth; be without acquisitiveness and possessiveness, a master of Self. (Even heaven belongs in the category of Nature).

For the brahmin who is wise, all the vedas are of as much use as a pool is in a place overflooded with water everywhere.

Yours is the right to action alone and never to the fruits thereof. Do not look for the fruit of action and do not be attached to inaction either.

Do your work, O Arjuna, being estblished in yoga, without attachment and being the same in success and failure; for evenmindedness (equanimity) is called yoga.

O Arjuna, far inferior is mere work to the yoga of understanding. Seek refuge in understanding; pitiful are they who seek the fruits of action.

He who has understanding shakes off good and evil even here. Strive therefore for yoga; yoga is skill in action.

The intelligent who have understanding renounce the fruit of action, and delivered from the bondage of birth they attain the state free from all anxiety.

When your understanding shall transcend the darkness of delusion, then you will be indifferent to what has been heard and is yet to be heard (scriptures which deal with law and rituals and the religion of heaven).

When your firm understanding shall remain fixed and unshaken in samadhi (the goal of yoga) without being perplexed by the scriptures (vedas) then you will attain to yoga.

MARKS OF A PERFECT YOGI

ARJUNA:

O Krishna! What are the marks of a person of steady wisdom, established in samadhi? How does a man of settled understanding speak, how does he sit and how does he walk?

KRISHNA:

When a person gives up all the desires of heart, O Arjuna, and is self-content in Self, then he is spoken of as a man of steady wisdom.

He who is not troubled in the midst of pain and is without craving amid pleasures and who is freed from attachment, fear and anger, he is called a sage of steady wisdom.

He who is without attachment everywhere and he who neither welcomes nor hates whatever falls to his lot, good or evil, his wisdom is steady.

And he who withdraws his senses from their objects like a tortoise retracts its limbs wholly into its shell, his wisdom is steady.

Sense-objects do not draw a person who is physically starved of them but the craving for them remains. But for him who has seen the Supreme even the craving for them ceases.

The impetuous senses, O Arjuna, carry off by force even the mind of a man who is discerning and striving for perfection.

Subduing them all, he who is devoted to Me (the Self) should remain established in yoga. He whose senses are under control, his wisdom is steady.

Attachment to sense objects arises in a person whose mind dwells on them. From attachment springs desire and from desires (thwarted) follows anger.

From anger comes delusion, from delusion loss of remembrance, from failure of remembrance loss of understanding and from loss of understanding, he perishes.

But a man of self-control who dwells on sense objects with the senses freed from their self-centered attachment and aversion and brought under self-rule, he attains peace of mind.

All his sorrows depart with the attainment of peace of mind. The understanding of a man whose mind is at peace is swiftly established in Self.

For the undisciplined there is no understanding, nor is there meditation for the undisciplined. And there is no peace for him who is without meditation. How can there be happiness for the unpeaceful?

The mind which follows the roving, self-centered senses steals away the understanding even as the wind carries away a boat on the waters.

Therefore, O Arjuna, he whose senses have been withdrawn fully from their objects, his wisdom is steady.

A man of self-control is awake in what is night for all other beings. That in which the beings are awake is night for the sage of vision.

As the ocean which remains ever motionless though being filled with waters which keep pouring into it, so also he into whom all desires vanish attains peace, but not the desirer of desires.

The man who lives and acts without attachment by renouncing all selfish desires and who is without the sense of me and mine, he attains peace.

This is the state of spiritual poise, O Arjuna, No one ever falls into delusion after attaining this. Established in it even at the final hour (of death) one achieves the supreme realization (brahma nirvana).

III
YOGA OF ACTION

KRISHNA:

In days of yore, O Arjuna, two roads to spiritual freedom have been shown by me, the path of knowledge for men of contemplation, and that of works for men of action.

A person does not achieve the state of inaction (calmness of contemplation) by just abstaining from action; nor does he attain perfection through renunciation alone.

None whosoever can remain inactive even for a moment. All are helplessly made to work by the forces of nature.

The deluded one who dwells inwardly on sense objects by restraining the senses of action is called a hypocrite.

But he who, O Arjuna, engages in the yoga of action with his senses disciplined by mind and in a spirit of detachment, he excels.

Do the work that is ordained; action is superior to inaction. Even your physical existence cannot be maintained without action.

Save work that is done as a sacrifice (i.e.,with understanding, in the spirit of yoga) this world creates the bondage of action. Therefore, O Arjuna, perform action without attachment.

In days of yore, the Lord of beings created men along with sacrifice (the obligation of service) and said: "By this you will grow and prosper, and let this fulfill all your desires.

You attend to the gods by this and let the gods serve you; thus serving each other,you will attain the Supreme good. (Society based on cooperation is the field where virtue and spirituality grow).

Therefore do always the work that is to be done without attachment. The person who performs work without attachment attains the Supreme.

It was by works that Janaka and others attained perfection. You should also work having in view the preservation of the world-order.

Whatever the great among men does, the others do the same; whatever standard he lays down,the world follows.

O Arjuna, for Me there is no obligation to work whatever in the three worlds, nor is there anything for me to have which I don't have, yet I am engaged in work.

As the ignorant, O Arjuna, act from attachment to work,so also the wise should work but without attachment, seeking to preserve the world-order.

The wise should not confuse the understanding of the ignorant who are attached to work, but he should set them to work by performing all actions in the spirit of yoga.

NATURE AND SELF

While all works are done by the gunas (principles, forces) of nature, the person deluded by the ego-sense thinks, "I am the doer."

But, O Arjuna, one who knows the truth of the distinction between the Self and the works done by nature (the gunas) understands that nature acts upon nature, and therefore does not become attached.

Those who are deluded by the gunas (principles) of nature become attached to their workings. But let not him who knows the whole truth unsettle those who are of poor understanding and know only little.

Even a man of wisdom acts in accordance with his nature. Creatures follow their dispositions. What can repression do?

Senses are self-centered in their relation of love and hate to their objects. Let no one be under their subjection, they are both his antagonists.

It is better to follow one's own nature though defective than to imitate another's virtue which is perfect. It is better to die by following one's own nature; it is perilous to imitate another's conduct.

The senses are beyond (the sense-objects), they say; the mind is beyond the senses; the intellect is beyond the mind, and He who stands above intellect is the Self.

Thus knowing the Self beyond intellect, and steadying the self by Self, O Arjuna, slay the enemy who is in the form of desire and difficult to get at.

IV

ANCIENT WISDOM AND DIVINE INCARNATION

KRISHNA:

I proclaimed the immortal truth of yoga to Vivasvan; Vivasvan spoke it to Manu, and Manu to Ikshvaku. (Vivasvan, Manu and Ikshvaku are traditional teachers of earlier ages.)

The royal sages knew this teaching handed down thus from one to another. Through long lapse of time, O Arjuna, this yoga was lost.

The same ancient yoga, the supreme secret, has today been proclaimed by Me to you, who are my devotee and also my friend.

ARJUNA:

Your birth was later, that of Vivasvan was earlier. How am I to know that you declared it to him in the beginning?

KRISHNA:

Many are my lives that are past, and yours also. I know them all but not you, O Arjuna.

Though I am unborn and imperishable and the Lord of all beings, I come into being (incarnate myself) dominating, through my own power of maya, Nature, which is an aspect (the dynamic) of my Self.

Whenever justice declines and injustice prevails, O Arjuna, then I create Myself (Step down on the stage of history as a Divine Incarnation).

For the protection of the good, for the destruction of the wicked and for the establishment of justice, I am born from age to age.

He who knows truly thus my divine birth and action, comes to Me, O Arjuna, transcending his egoistic existence.

In whatever way men approach Me, I appear to them in the same manner, O Arjuna! All men everywhere follow my path.

ACTION AND INACTION

Even the wise are bewildered about what is the right action and what is wrong. Therefore, I shall tell you what is right, knowing which you will be delivered from evil.

One has to understand what is right action and what is wrong and further what is inaction. The nature of work is hard to comprehend.

He who sees inaction in action (i.e., calm and detached inaction) and action in inaction, he is wise among men; he is a yogi and is the master of all action.

Without attachment to the fruits of work, ever content and without dependence, he does nothing although he is engaged in work.

The sacrifice of knowledge, O Arjuna, is superior to material sacrifice; for wisdom is the goal of all action. (Renunciation and freedom are essentially an attitude of mind.)

Know this truth through humility, inquiry and service. The wise, the seers of truth, will instruct you in wisdom.

There is nothing on earth so pure as wisdom. He who has attained perfection in yoga knows this himself in his heart in course of time.

A person of faith and devotion, who has controlled his senses gains wisdom, and having attained it,swiftly attains the Supreme Peace.

But the one who is ignorant and doubting and without faith, perishes. For the doubting soul there is neither this world, nor the other,nor any happiness.

V

TRUE RENUNCIATION

KRISHNA:

The renunciation of works and the yoga of action both lead to the Supreme Good. But of the two, the yoga of action is superior to its renunciation.

He who is dedicated to yoga, pure in spirit, master of self and who has conquered the senses and whose Self has become one with the Self of all, he is not bound by the works he does.

The Supreme Spirit does not create the agency and the works of individuals, nor the bondage to the fruits of work. It is Nature which originates all these.

The all-pervading Spirit accepts neither the sin nor the merit of any. Knowledge is covered by ignorance; the creatures are deluded thereby.

But for those whose ignorance has been destroyed by knowledge, wisdom lights up the Supreme Self like the sun.

The wise are samesighted toward the learned and humble brahmin, the cow, the elephant, the dog or even the outcaste.

Even here on earth they have conquered existence whose mind is established in sameness. The Spirit is without blemish and the same in all. Therefore they are established in the Spirit.

The sages whose impurities have been destroyed, whose doubts have been dispelled, who are self-possessed and who are engaged in doing good to all creatures, attain to the peace of nirvana in Brahman.

VI

TRUE YOGA

KRISHNA:

O Arjuna, know this, what they call renunciation is the yoga of action. No one who has not renounced the egotistic purpose ever becomes a yogi.

Save the self by the Self, never depress the Self. The Self alone is the friend of self and the Self alone is the enemy of self.

The Self is a friend of the Self for him who has conquered the self by the Self. But for one who is not Self-controlled the Self acts hostile like an enemy.

For man who is temperate in food and recreation and properly active and whose sleep and wakefulness are regulated — yoga removes all his suffering.

When the well-disciplined mind dwells in the Self alone without craving for anything at all, then is one said to have attained unity (with the Self.)

The yogi whose mind is controlled and concentrated on the Self is likened to a lamp which is without a flicker in a windless place.

Where the mind is at rest, stilled completely by the practice of yoga, where one takes delight in the Self, seeing the self by the Self; where one experiences the *ne plus ultra* of all happiness, perceptible to the subtle intellect and suprasensuous, and wherein established he does not ever slip from the truth; that, gaining which he does not regard any other gain superior to it, and established in which, he is not shaken by the greatest of pain — know that to be what is truly called yoga, the state above all misery. This yoga should be practiced steadfastly with a dauntless heart.

Supreme happiness comes to the yogi whose mind is peaceful, whose passions are at rest and who is stainless and one with the Divine.

He whose heart is established in yoga sees his Self in all beings and all beings in his Self, he is samesighted toward all.

He who sees Me everywhere and all in Me — I am not secret from him, nor is he from Me.

The yogi who is established in oneness and who worships Me abiding in all beings, he dwells in Me no matter what he does.

He who, O Arjuna, looks upon pleasure or pain in the same way everywhere as he does in himself is known as the perfect yogi.

ARJUNA:

O Krishna, the mind is restless and impetuous, stubborn and intractable; I regard it as difficult to control as the wind.

KRISHNA:

Doubtless, O Arjuna, the mind is restless and difficult to subdue. But it is controlled through practice and detachment.

IX
THE SPIRIT IS MORE THAN ITS MANIFESTATION

KRISHNA:

All this universe is pervaded by Me through my invisible Presence, all beings abide in Me, but I am not contained in them.

And yet the beings are not in Me, behold My divine mystery. My spirit which is the origin of all beings upholds them but does not dwell in them.

As the vast mass of air moving everywhere abides in space always, so also know that all beings dwell in Me.

All beings, O Arjuna, enter into My Nature at the end of a cycle; I project (create) them again at the beginning of another.

I am the Goal and the Sustainer, the Lord and the Witness, the Abode, the Refuge and the Friend (of all). I am the Beginning and the End, the Ground and the Resting Place and also the Imperishable Seed.

Whatever you do, whatever you eat, whatever you offer, whatever you give away, and whatever austerities you practice, O Arjuna, do that as an offering to Me.

I am the same to all beings. None is hateful or dear to Me. But those who worship Me with devotion, they are in Me and I am also in them.

X

SPIRIT AS THE SOURCE OF ALL

KRISHNA:

I am the origin of all, from Me everything comes into being. Knowing this, the wise who are of right understanding worship Me.

I, O Arjuna, am the Self, dwelling in the hearts of all. I am the beginning, the middle and the end of beings.

Of creations, I am the beginning, the end and also the middle, O Arjuna; of the sciences, I am the science of the Self and of those who debate, I am the dialetic.

Of letters, I am the letter A and of compounds, I am the dual; I am also the imperishable time; I am the ground of all everywhere.

I am the all-devouring Death and the origin of all that is going to be; of the feminine principles I am fame, prosperity, speech, memory, intelligence, patience and forgiveness.

Whatever is the seed of all beings that I am, O Arjuna; there is nothing among the moving and the unmoving which can exist without Me.

There is no end to My divine manifestations, O Arjuna. Whatever has so far been declared by Me only indicates their infinite variety.

Whatsoever there exists which is glorious, graceful and mighty know that to have originated from a fragment of My power.

But what, O Arjuna, is the need of your knowing this in detail. Pervading the whole universe with a fraction of My Being, I support and transcend all.

XI
THE COSMIC FORM

Arjuna wishes to see the Universal Form of the Divine, Krishna reveals it to him. After seeing it Arjuna speaks of other things.

You are the Imperishable, the Supreme Object of knowledge, you are the Ultimate Resting Place of the universe. You are the Immortal Guardian of the eternal law; you are the Primeval Spirit.

KRISHNA:
I am time, hoary and world-destroying, engaged here in gathering the beings. Even without you all these warriors standing in array in the opposing armies shall cease to be.

XII

Krishna describes the marks of a true yogi once again (see chapter II).

He has no enmity toward anyone but is friendly and compassionate to all. He is without the sense of me and mine (sense of egoism), and he is the same in pleasure and pain and is forgiving.

The yogi who is always content, self-controlled, of firm conviction, and whose mind and understanding are committed to me and who is My devotee is dear to Me.

He who neither troubles the world nor is troubled by it, who is free from elation and depression, from fear and anxiety is also dear to Me.

He who is above mirth and melancholy, who neither grieves nor desires, who is beyond good and evil and who is devoted is dear to Me.

He is the same toward friend or foe, the same in honor and dishonor, in cold and heat, in pleasure and pain and is without attachment.

He who is the same in praise and blame, restrained in speech, who is content with whatever comes his way, who is without a home, who is of steady conviction and who is devoted to Me, he is dear to Me.

But those faithful devotees who follow this immortal path of wisdom, holding Me as their supreme goal are exceedingly dear to Me.

XIII
THE FIELD, THE KNOWER AND DISCRIMINATION

KRISHNA:

This body, O Arjuna, is called the field and he who is the witness of this is called the knower of the field by men of perception (the body includes also mind, both being processes of nature. The witness is spirit or consciousness).

Know Me as the (one) witness in all the fields. The knowledge of the field and its knower (witness) I hold as the true knowledge.

KNOWLEDGE

Absence of pride and arrogance, non-injury, forgiveness, straightforwardness, service to the teacher, cleanliness, steadiness and self-control; non-attachment to sense-objects, absence of egoism and perception of the pains (of existence) of birth and death, decrepitude and disease; non-attachment, absence of blind attachment to son, wife, home and the like, and constant evenness of mind amid all happenings, desirable or undesirable; unfaltering devotion to Me through single-minded effort, love of solitude and distaste for crowds; constant knowledge of Self and perception of the subtle truths of existence — all this is declared to be knowledge; whatever is different from it is ignorance ("Virtue is Knowledge". Wisdom is character born of the perception of Truth).

I will describe that which is to be known and by knowing which one gains eternal life — the Supreme Brahman, which is without beginning and which is said to be neither existent nor non-existent.

With his hands and feet everywhere, eyes and face in every direction, and ears on all sides, He dwells, enveloping all.

He is without the senses though He seems to be tinged with their qualities; non-attached and yet upholding all, He is beyond the gunas (processes of nature) and yet he experiences them.

He is without and within all beings; he is moving and yet unmoving. So subtle to be perceived, he is far away and yet near.

Though He is indivisible yet He dwells as it were divided among beings. He is the origin, the support and the devourer (end) of all creatures.

Beyond darkness, He is the light of all lights. Knowledge, the object of knowledge and the goal to be known, He is seated in the hearts of all.

Know that both Spirit (purusha) and Nature (prakriti) are without beginning and know also that the gunas and their transformations are born of Nature (prakriti).

Nature is the cause of the body, the senses and egoism; Spirit is the cause of the experience of pleasure and pain.

The spirit dwelling in nature experiences the modes (gunas) born of it. Attachment to them is the cause of its birth (egoistic sense, embodiment) in good and evil wombs.

The Transcendent Spirit dwelling in the body is called the Seer, the Witness, the Supporter, the Experiencer, the Great Lord and the Supreme Self.

He who knows thus (the distinction of) the Spirit and Nature with its gunas never becomes embodied again (identified with body and mind i.e., limited by the processes of nature), no matter how he deports himself.

ROADS TO FREEDOM

Some perceive the Self in the self by the Self through meditation, others through the yoga of discrimination (philosophical analysis), and still others through the yoga of action.

Yet others, not knowing this, approach the goal through hearing from others; and even they, devoted to what they have heard, cross beyond death.

Whatever being comes into existence, moving or unmoving, O Arjuna, know that it is sprung from the union of the field and the witness of the field (Nature and Spirit).

He who sees the Supreme Lord abiding equally in all beings, imperishable while they perish, he indeed sees the truth.

Seeing the Lord present equally everywhere, he does not injure the Self by the self (does not harm others) and thus attains the supreme goal.

He who sees that all actions are done by nature alone and further that the Self is not the doer, he indeed sees the truth.

When he sees that the manifoldness of existence rests in unity and that it proliferates from it alone, then he attains Brahman.

Because the Imperishable Supreme Self is without beginning and without attributes (gunas), It, O Arjuna, neither acts nor is tainted though dwelling in the body.

As the all-pervading space is never tainted because of its subtlety, so also the Self dwelling in the body everywhere is not tainted.

As the solitary sun lights up the whole world, so does the witnessing spirit manifest the entire field.

Those who perceive thus with the eye of wisdom the distinction between the witnessing spirit (subject) and the field (object) and also the deliverance of beings from nature, they reach the Supreme.

XIV
THE DIVISION OF THE GUNAS

For the meaning of the gunas as the primary principles of Nature see the chapter on Nature. The gunas are secondarily used in an ethical sense to denote the qualities of lucidity and calmness (sattva), of passion and activity (rajas), of dullness and delusion (tamas). Here they are used in their ethical sense.

KRISHNA:

The three attributes of calmness, passion and dullness (sattva, rajas and tamas) are born of nature, they bind the imperishable spirit, O Arjuna, to the body. (Mental and physical states belong to nature, not to the witnessing spirit. In embodied existence the spirit becomes identified with them. This is its bondage.)

Of these, sattva, being pure, is illuminating and tranquil. It binds, O Arjuna, by attachment to happiness and to knowledge (science). (The sattva quality of calmness, idealism and intellectual knowledge is not devoid of ego-sense and therefore does not liberate a person).

Rajas (passion) is of the nature of impulse born of attachment and craving. It binds the embodied spirit by attachment to action.

Know tamas (dullness) to be born of ignorance; it deludes all embodied beings, O Arjuna, (by enveloping them) through forgetfulness, laziness and sleep.

Sattva attaches one to happiness, rajas to action, O Arjuna; but dullness, veiling knowledge, attaches one to forgetfulness.

When the powers of perception are heightened in all the gates of the body (senses), know then that sattva has increased.

When rajas dominates, O Arjuna, all these — greed, activity, ventures, unrest and craving arise.

And when tamas prevails these, O Arjuna, arise, namely, darkness, inactivity, forgetfulness, and delusion.

From sattva arises knowledge, from rajas greed and from tamas, forgetfulness, delusion and also ignorance.

When the seer perceives no other doer than the gunas and knows also that which is beyond the gunas, he attains unity with Me.

XV
THE COSMIC TREE

KRISHNA:

The imperishable ashvattha tree (peepal tree, i.e. the cosmic process) has its roots above and branches below. Its leaves are the Vedas, he who knows this is the Knower of the Vedas. (The world has its roots above in God. Veda is wisdom).

A fraction of Me has become the eternal soul in the world of living being and it draws unto itself the six senses including the mind, all of which are parts of Nature (prakriti).
(The empirical person is a mixture of spirit and nature.)

I am seated in the hearts of all; from Me come recollection and knowledge which destroys ignorance. I am the person to be known by all the Vedas; I am the author of the Vedanta and also the knower of the Vedas.

There are two persons in this world, the perishable and the imperishable; the perishable comprises all the beings, the imperishable is changeless.

But the Supreme Person is another, called the Transcendent Self, the Immortal Lord, who pervades and supports the three worlds.

Because I am above the perishable and higher even than the imperishable I am celebrated in the world and in the Vedas as the Supreme Person.

XVI
THE DIVINE AND THE DEMONIAC NATURES

KRISHNA:

Fearlessness, purity of mind, dedication to knowledge and meditation, charity, self-control, sacrifice, study of scriptures, austerity and straightforwardness, non-injury, truth, absence of anger, renunciation, tranquillity, tolerance, compassion to living beings, greedlessness, gentleness, modesty and steadiness, spiritedness, forgiveness, fortitude, purity, non-enmity, absence of arrogance

—these are, O Arjuna, the endowments of one born with the divine nature.

Bluster, pride, arrogance, anger, rudeness and ignorance—these, O Arjuna, are the traits of one born with the demoniac nature.

The demoniac know neither the path of action nor that of renunciation. Neither purity, nor good conduct, nor truth is found in them.

The world, they proclaim, is without truth and has no other basis. It is born of chance, and what else can it exist for, except pleasure?

Holding to this view, these lost souls of little understanding appear in the world as its enemies, violent in their deeds and bent upon its destruction.

Cherishing insatiable desire, full of bluster, hyprocrisy and arrogance, these men of impure motives pursue evil ends through delusion.

Given to endless worries until death, regarding the enjoyment of pleasure as the highest end and cocksure that this is all;

Chained by a million bonds of desire and given over to lust and rage, they struggle by corrupt means to make piles of fortune for the enjoyment of pleasure.

"This I have gained today; this other desire I shall satisfy, this wealth is mine and I shall also have more;

This foe I have slain, I shall slay the others also; I am the lord and the enjoyer; I have success and power; I am happy;

I am wealthy and high-born. Who else is there like unto me? I shall endow and give and rejoice." thus they brag deluded by ignorance.

Bewildered by endless schemes, entangled in the meshes of delusion and addicted to pleasure, they sink into hellish existence.

Self-conceited, stubborn, intoxicated with the pride and arrogance of wealth, they sacrifice (make endowments) only in name with ostentation and impropriety.

Given over to egotism, violence, arrogance, lust and rage these malicious people hate Me who dwells in all bodies, theirs and others.

These dregs of men, pitiless, evil and hateful—I hurl them over and over again into cycles of demoniac existence.

He who follows the promptings of desire without regard to spiritual law, he attains neither perfection, nor happiness, nor the supreme goal.

Therefore, let the scripture be your authority in determining what is right or not right to do. You should act in the world following what the scripture declares to be according to law.

XVII
FAITH AND AUSTERITY

KRISHNA:

The faith of every individual, O Arjuna, is in accordance with his nature. A man is made by his faith; whatever his faith is so is he.

Dedication of wealth and service (sacrifice) which is according to spiritual law by those who desire no reward and who dedicate from a sense of obligation is sattvika in character (i.e., just and right and good).

But that which is offered in the hope of reward or for the sake of display know that, O Arjuna, to be rajasika (passionate) or tainted in character.

The worship of the gods, the twice-born, the teachers and the wise men and the practice of purity, straightforwardness, continence and non-violence are said to be the penance of the body.

Use of words which do not aggravate, which are true, pleasant and beneficial, and the regular recitation of scriptures are called the penance of speech.

Serenity of mind, gentleness, silence, self-control and purity of motive are called the penance of mind.

This threefold austerity practiced with supreme faith and fervor by men who are disciplined and without desire for reward is said to be sattvika in character (i.e. the best or highest).

The austerity which is practiced with the object of gaining respect, honor and reverence and with ostentation is said to be rajasika (tainted) in nature; it is unstable and fleeting.

The austerity which is performed stupidly, causing self-torture or for the sake of destroying others, is said to be tamasika (stupid or blind) in kind.

The gift which is made from a sense of duty to one from whom no help has been received or is expected and which is given in the right time, the right place and to the right person is called the sattvika (best) gift.

But the gift which is made in return for the help received or in the hope of future gain and which is given grudgingly is known to be the rajasika (tainted) gift.

And the gift which is given at the wrong time, the wrong place, to the wrong person without grace and with contempt is said to be the tamasika (lowest, stupid) gift.

XVIII
WORK AND RENUNCIATION

KRISHNA:

Giving up of work that ought to be done is not right; its renunciation through delusion is said to be tamasika (stupid).

But, O Arjuna, he who performs the work that should be done, renouncing attachment and its fruit, his renunciation is considered sattvika (highest).

The wise man of true renunciation, who is established in truth and whose doubts have been dispelled, neither hates work which is unpleasant nor is attached to action that is pleasant.

KNOWLEDGE

The knowledge by which the Imperishable Being is seen as one and undivided among all the beings which are separate, know that knowledge to be sattvika (the best).

The knowledge which sees the variety of existences as multiple and separate everywhere, know that knowledge to be rajasika (tainted) in character.

It is better to follow one's nature though defective than to imitate another's virtue however meritorious. One does not incur evil by doing work ordained by one's nature.

One should not, O Arjuna, give up the work which is according to one's nature though it is defective. All actions are covered with defects like fire by smoke.

The Lord dwells in the hearts of all, O Arjuna, making them move like puppets mounted on a machine.

Take refuge in Him in every way, O Arjuna. By His grace you will attain the supreme peace and the eternal abode.

Abandoning all rules, take refuge in Me alone. Do not sorrow, I will emancipate you from all evils.

CONCLUSION

Sanjaya (the speaker who reports the dialogue between Krishna and Arjuna) concludes:

Where there is Krishna, the Lord of yoga and Arjuna, the archer, there I am sure will always be fortune, victory, progress and unfailing justice. (Spiritual vision and power are the conditions of a just and progressive social order.)

OTHER SELECTIONS

BELOW ARE A FEW selections from later sources including those of our time.

Harder than adamant and softer than flowers are the hearts of men of extraordinary character.

Bhavabhuti (4th Cent.)

World-Teacher and Lord of the universe! In my meditations I have imagined you who is formless as having form; in my hymns I have denied your inexpressible nature; and by my pilgrimages I have disavowed your all-pervasiveness—forgive me, Ruler of all, these three faults of mine due to my human limitations.

Sanskrit Prayer

"This is my own, that is a stranger," is the calculation of the narrow-hearted; to the large-hearted the whole world is kin.

Ancient Sanskrit saying

Uncleansed desires create bondage, purified desires give liberation.

Yoga Vashishtha (Hindu scripture)

I salute the supreme teacher, the Truth, whose nature is Bliss, who is the giver of the highest happiness, who is pure wisdom, who is beyond all dualities and infinite like the sky, who is beyond words, who is one and eternal, pure and still, who is beyond all change and phenomena, and who is the silent witness to all our thoughts and emotions — I salute Truth, the supreme teacher.

From popular Sanskrit hymn

I close not my eyes, stop not my ears, nor torment my body.

But every path I then traverse becomes a path of pilgrimage,
    whatever work I engage in becomes service.

The simple consummation is the best.

> *Kabir (Medieval Hindu Saint—16th cent.)*

All see the Eternal One, but only the devotee, in his solitude, recognizes him.

> *Kabir*

I have known in my body the sport of the universe; I have escaped from the
    illusion of this world.

The inward and the outward are become as one sky, the Infinite and the
    finite are united; I am drunken with the sight of this all!

This light of thine fulfils the universe; the lamp of love that burns on the
    salver of knowledge.

Kabir says: There error cannot enter, and the conflict of life and death is felt
    no more.

> *Kabir*

All things are created by the Om;
The love-form is His body.
He is without form, without quality, without decay.
Seek thou union with Him!
But that formless God takes a thousand forms in the eyes of His creatures;
He is pure and indestructible,
His form is infinite and fathomless,
He dances in rapture, and waves of form arise from His dance.
The body and the mind cannot contain themselves, when they are touched
    by His great joy.
He is immersed in all consciousness, all joys and sorrows;
He has no beginning and no end;
He holds all within His bliss.

> *Kabir*

When He himself reveals himself,
Brahman brings into manifestation
That which can never be seen.

As the seed is in the plant, as the shade is in the tree; as the void is in the
   sky, as infinite form are in the void—
So from beyond the Infinite, the Infinite comes; and from the Infinite the
   finite extends.
The creature is in Brahma, and Brahma is in the creature; they are never
   distinct, yet ever united.
He himself is the tree, the seed, and the germ.
He himself is the flower, the fruit, and the shade.
He himself is the sun, the light, and the lighted.
He himself is Brahma, creature, and Maya.
He himself is the manifold form, the infinite space;
He is the breath, the word, and the meaning
He himself is the limit and the limitless; and beyond both the limited and
   the limitless is He, the Pure Being.
He is the Imminent Mind in Brahma and in the creature.

Kabir

The Supreme Self is seen within the soul,
The Point is seen within the Supreme Self,
And within the Point, the reflection is seen again.
Kabir is blest because he has this supreme vision!

Kabir

Within the Supreme Brahma, the worlds are being told like beads;
Look upon that rosary with the eyes of wisdom.

Kabir

Between the poles of the Conscious and the Unconscious, there has the mind
   made a swing;
Thereon hang all beings and all worlds, and that swing never ceases its sway.
Millions of beings are there, the sun and the moon in their courses are there;
Millions of ages pass, and the swing goes on.
All swing! the sky and the earth and the air and the water; and the Lord
   Himself taking form;
And the sight of this has made Kabir a servant.

Kabir

All the world is the Veda, all creations Koran. Why read paper scriptures,
   O Rajja?
Gather ever fresh wisdom from the universe.
The eternal wisdom shines within the concourse of the millions of Humanity.
                                                    Rajjab (Med. Hindu Saint)

Listen, O brother man,
Above all Man is true
There is no truth higher.
                        Chandidas (Mystic Bengali poet; 17th cent.)

"And lo! the whole scene, doors, windows, the temple itself vanished.... It
seemed as if nothing existed any more. Instead I saw an ocean of spirit,
boundless, dazzling. In whatever direction I turned great luminous waves
were rising. They bore down upon me with a loud roar; as if to swallow me
up. In an instant they were upon me. They broke over me, they engulfed me.
I was suffocated. I lost all outer consciousness and I fell.... How I passed the
day and the next I know not. Round me rolled an ocean of ineffable joy..."
                                                    Sri Ramakrishna

"When I was eighteen, a sudden spring breeze of religious experience for the
first time came to my life and passed away leaving in my memory a direct
message of spiritual reality. One day while I stood watching at early dawn,
the sun sending out its rays from behind the trees, I suddenly felt as if some
ancient mist had in a moment lifted from my sight, and the morning light
on the face of the world revealed an inner radiance of joy. The invisible
screen of the commonplace was removed from all things and all men, and
their ultimate significance was intensified in my mind; and this is the definition of beauty. That which was memorable in this experience was its human
message, the sudden expansion of my consciousness in the super-personal
world of man. The poem I wrote on the first day of my surprise was named:
"The Awakening of the Waterfall." The waterfall, whose spirit lay dormant
in its ice-bound isolation, was touched by the sun and, bursting in a cataract
of freedom, it found its finality in an unending sacrifice, in a continual union
with the sea. After four days the vision passed away, and the lid hung down
upon my inner sight. In the dark, the world once again put on its disguise
of the obscurity of an ordinary fact.

"When I grew older and was employed in a responsible work in some villages, I took my place in a neighborhood where the current of time ran slow

and joys and sorrows had their simple and elemental shades and lights. The day, which had its special significance for me, came with all its drifting trivialities of the commonplace life. The ordinary work of my morning had come to its close, and before going to take my bath I stood for a moment at my window, overlooking a market place on the bank of a dry river bed, welcoming the first flood of rain along its channel. Suddenly I became conscious of a stirring of soul within me. My world of experience in a moment seemed to become lighted, and facts that were detached and dim found a great unity of meaning. The feeling which I had was like that which a man, groping through a fog without knowing his destination, might feel when he suddenly discovers that he stands before his own house."

Rabindranath Tagore

Let me not pray to be sheltered from dangers but to be fearless in facing them.
Let me not beg for the stilling of my pain but for the heart to conquer it.
Let me not look for allies in life's battlefield but to my own strength.
Let me not crave in anxious fear to be saved but hope for the patience to win
  my freedom.
Grant me that I may not be a coward, feeling your mercy in my success alone;
  but let me find the grasp of your hand in my failure.

The Devil's wares are expensive.
God's gifts are without price.

I am able to love my God
because he gives me freedom to deny him.

God honored me with his fight when I was rebellious;
He ignored me when I was languid.

The man proud of his sect
thinks that he has the sea
ladled into his private pond.

My faith in Truth, my vision of the perfect,
help thee, Master, in thy creation.

The fire restrained in the tree fashions flowers,
Released from bonds, the shameless flame dies in barren ashes.

Some have thought deep
and expressed the meaning of thy truth and they are great;
I have listened to catch the music of thy play and I am glad.

Mistakes live in the neighborhood of truth and therefore delude us.

Day with its glare of curiosity makes the stars disappear.
The sky, though holding in his arms his bride, the earth,
is ever immensely away.

The world is the everchanging foam
that floats on the surface of a sea of silence.

Faith is the bird that feels the light
and sings when the dawn is still dark.

Leaves are masses of silence,
round flowers which are their words.

Let our life be beautiful like summer flowers.
And death glorious like autumn leaves.

Rabindranath Tagore

"I do dimly perceive that whilst everything around me is ever-changing, ever-dying, there is underlying all that change a Living Power that is changeless, that holds all together, that creates, dissolves and recreates. That informing Power of Spirit is God; and since nothing else that I see merely through the senses can or will persist, He alone is... All else is illusion—Maya. We are not, He alone is."

M. K. Gandhi

"Only those thoughts are true, the opposite of which is also true in its own time and application. Indisputable dogmas are the most dangerous kind of falsehoods."

Sri Aurobindo

There is neither the sun, nor the lovely moon, nor a star.
In the infinite space floats shadow-like the image universe.
In the primeval mind the world-process floats;
It floats and sinks and rises again in the ceaseless stream of "I am."
Slowly the throng of shadows depart and merge in the primal abode.
Now flows unbroken the feeling of pure "I" and "I" alone.
That flow also ceases, void merges in the Void.
Beyond the reach of speech and mind,
He knows whose heart knows.

Swami Vivekananda

Man wants to measure the ocean of Truth with the cup of his mind.

Life's end is not in a perfection that is final,
but in a completion that is endless.

The glare of a little sun hides the giant luminaries of the heavens, but the darkness of night reveals their splendor in the depths of interstellar space. The clamor of the phantom ego obscures the immortal Truth of Spirit, but the stillness of meditation manifests Its eternal glory in the immensity of a boundless Silence.

Man is born in chains but struggles through history toward the
Freedom beyond.

Life is a great gift to be lived,
Laying waste to our soul is not peace.

Truth is more than consistency,
Beauty is more than harmony,
And love is more than law.

S. K. Majumdar

A Marriage Benediction:

May these two young hearts be united one to the other like flower and its perfume, like flute and its melody; may they have many summers of sweet love and happiness; may they bring forth children and grandchildren; may they in the autumn of life ripen through service into the serenity of Spirit; and may they at the end of their days break all mortal bonds and encounter the Great Unknown with fearless heart.

Truth is revealed in communication,
Perfect communication is achieved in Silence.

S. K. Majumdar

SELECT BIBLIOGRAPHY

SELECT BIBLIOGRAPHY

THE YOGA SUTRAS OF PATANJALI with the commentary of Vyasa have long been regarded as the classical yoga texts, but as I have mentioned earlier, Patanjali represents one school, and his views are not to be regarded as representing the broad tradition of yoga. Patanjali's work is however the first available systematic presentation of yoga principles and practices and has been hailed as authoritative by a long line of writers who have commented and annotated upon it. The study of this book is a must for all students of yoga.

Unfortunately neither Patanjali nor his commentator Vyasa can be properly understood without extra help. The available English translations of these works are very often confusing, full of misinterpretations and lacking in understanding of key concepts. The only good and reliable translation and exposition, done by the late Swami Hariharananda Aranya, is in Bengali.

For English readers who do not know Sanskrit or Bengali the two following translations and commentaries can be recommended with some reservations:

1. RAJA YOGA by Swami Vivekananda
2. YOGA SUTRAS OF PATANJALI with the commentary of Vyasa: translated by Ganganath Jha

Works on yoga in English are numerous, but the best two expositions of Patanjali are:

1. A STUDY OF YOGA by Jnajneshwar Ghosh
2. YOGA AS RELIGION AND PHILOSOPHY by S. N. Dasgupta

The following are recommended for an understanding of the broad and living tradition of yoga:

1. THE PRINCIPAL UPANISHADS: Edited and translated by S. Radhakrishnan
2. THE BHAGAVAD GITA: Edited and translated by S. Radhakrishnan
3. RELIGION OF MAN by Rabindranath Tagore
4. SADHANA by Rabindranath Tagore
5. COLLECTED POEMS AND PLAYS by R. Tagore
6. POEMS OF KABIR: Translated by R. Tagore
7. LIFE DIVINE by Sri Aurobindo
8. HATHA YOGA by Shyam Sundar Goswami
9. YOGA ASANAS AND PRANAYAMA by Swami Kuvalayananda
10. WESTERN PSYCHOTHERAPHY AND HINDU SADHANA by Hans Jacobs

GLOSSARY OF
SANSKRIT WORDS

GLOSSARY OF SANSKRIT WORDS

Abhaya	Fearless, Fearlessness
Abhyasa	Practice
Aditya	The Sun God
Ahamkara	Ego sense; dynamic ego
Ahimsa	Non-injury, Love, Compassion
Ajna	Command, A center of spiritual consciousness (chakra) located between the eyebrows
Ambhrina	Name of a vedic sage.
Anahata	Name of a chakra, or center of spiritual consciousnes in the heart
Anubhava Prakasha	Name of hatha yoga book
Aparoksha	Immediate
Aranyaka	Forest treatise containing philosophical reflections.
Ardhamatsyendrasana	The side spinal twist posture
Arsha	Made or founded by the sage
Arya	Noble
Asamprajnata samadhi	Non-cognitive i.e. objectless awareness.
Asmita	Pure "I" sense, pure ego
Aswins	Vedic gods, twins
Atharvaveda	One of the four vedas
Atman, Atma	Self, soul individual and universal
Atmarati	One who takes delight in self.
Atmanam Biddhi	Know Thyself
Atmastha	Self-established
Avyakta	The unmanifest
Avidya	Ignorance, Illusion, maya
Bandha	Lock, contraction
Bhakti	Devotion, Love
Bhakti Yoga	Way of union with the Divine through love and devotion
Bhandara	Feast
Bhastrika	Bellows, breathing
Bhujangasna	Serpent Posture

Bhuma	The Infinite
Bhuta	Become, the sensible, element
Brahman	The Vast, Spirit, Reality
Brahmana	Vedic Ritualistic works; priest
Brahmalveshma	The Citadel of Brahman or Spirit; the heart center (chakra)
Brahma Sutras	An early philosophical work on the teachings of the Upanishad in the form of aphorisms like the Yoga Sutras of Patanjali
Brihadaranyaka Upanishad	An Upanishad
Buddha, The	Enlightened
Buddha hridaya	Heart of the Buddha
Buddhi	Intellect; the Pure Ego or Asmita
Chakra	Center, Center of spiritual consciousness
Chitra	Name of a nerve current
Dahara pundarika	The subtle lotus of the heart
Darshana	Vision, perception, philosophy
Dhanurasama	Bow posture
Dharana	The first stage of yogic concentration
Dharma	Law, Nature, Religion
Dhyana	Concentration, mediation
Dhauti	Cleansing
Drashta	The seer, pure subject, spirit
Drishya	The seen, the object, nature
Ekagra	One-pointed
Ghatastha Yoga	Yoga of the physical body, physical discipline
Gheranda Samhita	Name of a yoga book
Goraksha Samhita	A yoga book
Gita, The	The song. A practical composition of 700 verses forming part of the Hindu epic the Mahabharata. It is one of the basic scriptures of the Hindus.
Ha	A symbol for the energy-conserving principle, also called the sun principle.
Halasana	The plow pose
Hatha Yoga	Yoga of physical and mental health.
Hathadipika	A book on hatha yoga
Ida	A nerve current
Indriya	Sense function, sense organ
Ishwara	The Divine as the Ruler of Cosmos; the personal aspect of the Godhead

Jalandhara bandha	A special type of contraction in hatha yoga
Japa	Repetition of sacred words and syllables
Jnana	Knowledge
Jnanayoga	The Way of philosophical analysis and discrimination
Kapalabhati	Bellows breathing
Karma	Action, result of action, habit, tendency, etc.
Karma yoga	The way of action
Kathopanishad	The name of an Upanishad
Kena Upanishad	Name of an Upanishad
Kundalini	The coiled serpent power; the dormant spiritual energy
Laya	Mergence
Laya Yoga	The method of attaining samadhi or super-consciousness through meditation on sound vibration.
Mahabharata, The	A Hindu Epic (1500 B.C.) in Sanskrit.
Mahabhuta	The gross sensible
Mahadeva	The great god, Shiva
Mahamudra	The great pose
Mahat	The Great; The Cosmic Ego
Manas	Mind
Manana	Reflection, reasoning
Manipura	The center of spiritual consciousness located along the spine and against the navel.
Mantra	Verse, sacred word, word capable of rousing spiritual energy.
Mantra Yoga	Method of attaining spiritual realization through the repetition of sacred words or syllables.
Matsyasana	The Fish posture
Mayurasana	The Peacock pose
Mitra	A vedic god
Mudha	Stupid, dull
Mulabandha	The root contraction
Muladhara	The center of spiritual consciousness at the base of the spine.
Mundaka Upanishad	Name of an Upanishad
Nachiketas	A vedic brahmin boy
Nama	Name

Nauli	Isolation of abdominal recti
Neti	Nasal cleansing
Nididhyasana	Meditation
Nidra	Sleep
Nirodha	Stoppage
Niruddha	Arrested
Nirvana	Blowing out; Superconsciousness or Samadhi
Nirvikalpa	Without any mental formation
Nirvikalpa Samadhi	The highest state of meditation
Niyama	Rule of conduct
Om	The most sacred sound symbol of the Divine among the Yogis.
Rajas	The dynamic principle of nature; one of the three gunas.
Rasa	Delight
Rig Veda	One of the four vedas
Rita	Truth, order, law
Rudra	A vedic god; shiva
Rupa	Form
Sahasrara	The thousand-petalled lotus; the center of spiritual consciousness (chakra) in the top brain.
Samaveda	One of the four vedas
Samadhi	Superconsciousness
Samhita	A collection
Samkhya Yoga	Yoga of knowledge, yoga of philosophical analysis
Samskara	Impression, habit, tendency, the unconscious factors
Samyama	Perfect control; a form of concentration
Sanatana dharma	The Perennial Religion
Sarvangasana	The pan-physical pose; the shoulder stand
Sat	The Real; the true
Sattva	Being, one of the gunas, the principle of intelligibility in nature.
Satyakama	The name of a vedic student
Savikalpa samadhi	Determinate or cognitive superconscious experience
Shalabhasana	The lotus pose
Shanti	Peace
Shatkarma	The six cleansing techniques of hatha yoga

Shavasana	The corpse pose
Shirshasana	The head stand
Shiva	The Divine in the aspect of the Good
Shivasamhita	A book on hatha yoga
Shravana	Hearing
Shushumna	The central line of spiritual current in the spine on the awakening of the dormant spiritual energy called the kundalini.
Shvetashwatara Upanishad	Name of a vedic Upanishad
Siddhasana	The perfect pose
Sindhu	The Indus river
Smriti	Memory
Soma	The moon; a vedic drink
Sukhasana	Easy or happy pose
Suptavajrasana	The dormant pelvic pose
Svadhishthana	The second of the six centers of spiritual consciousness located above the genitals.
Svadlhyaya	Study or recitation of scripture.
Tamas	Darkness; the dark or the conservative principle in nature, the principle of inertia, of resistance, of mass.
Tanmatra	"That Alone"; the infrasensible particles or units of energy; the subtle activity behind sensible qualities that is felt in advanced concentration; a stage of development of nature prior to sensible phenomena.
Tattva	"Thatness"; a principle, a state or stage of development in nature.
Tha	The moon principle or the energy storing process in the body.
Trataka	Fixed gazing on specially chosen objects for concentration and eye exercise.
Trikonasana	The triangle posture
Upanishad	The wisdom section of the vedic literature; the mystery learning.
Vairagya	Detachment, non-attachment
Vajra	Name of a nerve current
Vak	A vedic goddess
Varuna	A vedic god (buranos)
Vasu	A vedic god

Veda — Knowledge, sacred literature of the Hindus

Vedanta — End portion of the Vedas, Upanishads, philosophy of the Upanishads.

Vikalpa — Intellectual construction, mental formation

Vikriti — Transformation

Vikshipta — Scattered, restless

Viparya — Error

Vira — Man, hero

Vishuddha — Pure; the center of spiritual consciousness located in the throat area.

Vishvakosha — Name of a hatha yoga book

Vyakta — Manifest

Yama — Control, restraint, ethical discipline. Also the king of death, a vedic god.

Yoga — Harnessing; union; method of union; way; self knowledge and means of self realization.

INDEX

INDEX

Abdomen, 143, 144, 146, 178-179
Abdominal recti muscles, 178-180
Abdomino-recti muscle control, 178-180
Abhyasa, 67, 191
Action, 34, 95
Adhyatma Yoga, 22
Agnisara, 175
Ahimsa, 221
Ajna chakra, 207
Alimentary system, 174, 175
Alms house, 119-120
Amarnath, cave of, 127
American Indians, 220
Amitabha Buddha, 44
Anahata chakra, 207
Anal contraction, 174
Animal, the, 35
Anubhava Prakasha, 138
Aparoksha, 74
Apathy, 226
Apollonian dictum, 27
Aranyakas, 21
Ardha Matsyendrasana, 158-159
Aristotle, 26
Arjuna, 41, 190-191
Arsha dharma, 47
Art, 65
Arthakriyakaritva, 88
Arthritis, 110, 213
Art of Healing Breath, The, 107-108
Aryans, 21, 24
Aryan truths, 44
Asamprajnata samadhi, 58-59

Asana, 105
Asanas. See also Poses, Postures.
Asceticism, 36-37
— and self-discipline, 127-128
— and yoga, 127-128
Ashramas, 116-117
Asmita, 80-81
Astrology, 94
Atman, 67
Atmarati, 74
Atmastha, 74
Austerity, 224
Autarch, 27
Avidya, 44, 76-77
Avyakta, 79, 80, 82
Awareness, 58, 66-67
— levels of, 206
— mystic, 220-221
— principle of, 79
— pure, 188, 193

Back, the, 143, 146
Back stretching pose, 146
Bacon, Francis, 56
Bakaki Bharati, 102, 103
Bandha, 105
Bandhas, 173-174
Basic truths, four, 44
Bauls, 65
Bears, Himalayan, 118-119
Being, 61
— freedom of, 95
— mystery of, 227

Bellows breathing, 135
Berdyaev, 104
Beyond, the, 77
Bhagavad Gita. See Gita, The.
Bhakti, 54, 72
Bhakti Yoga, 54, 56
Bhandara, 121
Bhang, 220
Bhastrika, 135
Bhujangasana, 143
Bhuma, 34. *See also* Infinite, the.
Bhutas, 81
Bible, The, 29, 43
Biblical belief, 14
Blood, purity of, 181
Bodhidharma, 64
Body, the, 146
— and mind, 218-219
— and Spirit, 214, 216
Bombay, 102
Bow posture, 145, 183
Brahmabeshma, 207
Brahman, 32
Brahman, citadel of, 207
Brahmanadi, 209
Brahmanas, 21
Brahma Sutras, 74
Brahmavidya, 23
Bread, 122
Breath control, 100, 160, 198-199.
   See also Hatha Yoga.
Breathing, 107-109, 140. *See also* Pra-
   nayama.
— abdominal, 130-131
— absolute suspension, 134
— bellows, 135
— collarbone, 133
— complete, 133-134
— complete, for women, 134
— exercises, 130, 200-204

— and physiological processes, 199
— and psyche, 109
— and psychic conditions, 199
— ribcage, 131-132
— Ujjayai, 136
Brown, Yeats, 103
Buddha, 22, 39, 43, 64, 115, 220
Buddha, *Amitabha,* 44
Buddha, heart of the, 221
Buddhahridaya, 221
Buddhi, 80-81
Buddhism, 43
— and karma, 90
— Mahayana, 44, 64-65
— Sanskrit, 44
— and Yoga, 43-45
— Zen, 189

Calcutta, 103
Camel pose, the, 151
Cancer, 108
Celibacy, 36-37
Centers of consciousness, 204
Central nauli, 180
Chakras, 204, 206-207, 209
Chakrasana, 150
Charana, 105
Charvakas, 73
Chhandogya Upanishad, 31, 45
Childbirth, 107
Chit, 78
Chitra, 206
Christianity, 43
Christianity, from Indian sources, 29
Civilization, contemporary, 28
Civilization, Greek, 27-29
Cleanliness, 110-111
Cleansing methods, 111, 174-181

Cobra posture, 143, 145, 183
Colonic auto-lavage, 176-177
Compassion, 224
Concentration, 58-59, 67, 188, 190, 210, 211
— and samadhi, 67
— stages of, 220
Conduct, rules of, 192
Consciousness, 68, 77, 83
— centers of, 204
— Cosmic, 39
— metempiric, 80
— pure, 12, 78, 80
Contemplation, 34, 95. See also meditation.
Cosmic Mind, 83
Cosmic Person, 198
Cosmic Self, 90
Cosmos, the, 77
Creation, 82
Creative power, 14
Creativity, 38
Culture, Upanishadic, 27-28

Dahara pundarika, 207
Darshana, 25-26. See Perception.
Davy, Sir Humphrey, 220
Dead pose, 172-173, 183
Dechanet, Father, 104
Democritus, 25
Dental Care, 175-176
Detachment, 191-192
Devotion, 54. See also Bhakti.
Dhanurasana, 145
Dharali, 124
Dharma, arsha, 47
Dharma, manava, 47
Dharma, sanatana, 47
Dharana, 188
Dhatura, 220

Dhauti, 174, 175
Dhyana, 54, 64, 188, 189, 199
Dhyana yoga, 54
Diaphragm, 178-179
Dieting, 128-129
Disciplines, 127-128
Disciplines, spiritual, 68-69
Discontents of Civilization, The, 31
Discrimination, 67
Diseases, cure through exercise, 184
Diseases, emotional origin of, 213
Divine, the 13, 41, 71, 196, 197
— in man, 35
— Idea, 196
— Intelligence, 196
— Person, 196, 197
— meditation on, 195
— Principle, 224
— Ruler, the, 198
— meditation on, 197
Dream experience, meditation on, 211
Drishya Prakriti, 78
Drug experience, 193
Drugs, and health, 219-221
— and mental health, 217-221
— and mental states, 217-218
— and Samadhi, 217-221
— and spiritual illumination, 217
— and tranquillity, 217-220
— use of, 218-221
Dukes, Sir Paul, 103-104
Dvijas, 21
Dvijatis, 37

East and West, meaning of, 28
Easy posture, 179, 200, 203
Ego, 73, 196
Egotism, 224

Egypt, 25
Egyptians, 25
Ekagra, 67-68
Empedocles, 25
Encyclopaedia of Indian Physical Culture, 105
Endocrine development, 182
Endocrine degeneration, 181
Enema, 177
Energies of Men, The, 104
Energy, 91
Enlightenment, 64. See also Satori.
Epinomis, 29
Essence, 40
Essenes, the, 29
Ethics, 41, 192
— as rules of conduct, 221-225
Ethical conduct, 222
Eusebius, 27
Evolution, 69-72
— order of, 81
Exercise, benefits of, 184
— for women, 156
— wrong method of, 111
— yoga posture, 130
Exercises, breathing, 130, 200-204
— order of, 182-183
— yoga, 129
— See also Breathing; Poses; Postures.
Existence, levels of, 87
Existentialism, 60-64
— in relation to Yoga and Zen, 60-64

Faith, 61-62, 63, 72
— in healing, 219
Faith healing, 214
Fasting, 112, 114, 128-129
Feelings, meditation and, 226-227
— pseudomystical, 220
Fish, 115

Fish posture, 149, 183
Five infrasensibles, 81
Five sensibles, 81
Food, a healthy diet of, 128
— and city dwellers, 122
— habits, 112
— for mendicants, 120-121
— of ascetics, 121-122
Freedom, 69-70, 72, 85, 87, 95, 225
— human, 89
— spiritual, 69-70
Freud, Sigmund, 31

Gandhi, 42
Ganges, the, 116-117, 120, 122-123
Gangotri, 124-127
Gazing, technique of, 180-181
Gerontology, 113
Ghatastha Yoga, 100
Gheranda Samhita, 101-102, 138
Gitanjal, 102
Gita, The, 23-24, 34, 36, 41-47, 63, 78, 82, 95, 190, 195, 198, 222, 223
Glands, 110
— and youthfulness, 181-182
God, 33, 48
Gonadal efficiency, 182
Good, absolute, 222-223
Goraksha Samhita, 101-102, 173
Goswami, Shyam Sundar, 102-103
Great pose, 160
Greek(s), 24-25
— civilization, 27-29
— and Hindu, as one people, 26
— reason, 14
Guilt, sense of, 223
Gunas, the, 78-80
Gune, J. G., 102
Gurdjieff, Georges Ivanovitch, 104
Guzrat, 102

Ha, the, 100
Halasana, 148
Hall, H. R., 25
Happiness, 75-76, 86, 93, 201
Haridas, 208-209
Harshil, 123
Hatha, definition of, 54
Hatha Dipika, 101-102, 138
Hatha Yoga, 54-56, 99, 103
— and spirituality, 209
— cleansing techniques of, 111
— history of, 101
Headknee bend, 156, 183
Head stand, 154, 183
Health, 99
— and meditation, 213-215
Heart and mind, as one, 196
Heart, the, 195-196, 202
Heart center, 207
Heart disease, 109-110, 213
Heraclitus, 25
Herbs, aromatic, 126
Hindu, derivation of the word, 47
Hinduism, 36, 42-43
— and Yoga, 46-47
Hindus, 47
Hips, the, 144
Hip stand, 157
Holy men, 117
Holy places, 215
Horoscopes, 94
Humanistic concern, 75
Human suffering, 44
Hume, David, 72-73
Huxley, Aldous, 35

"I", Cosmic, 207
Ida, 206, 209-210
Ideal, personal, 195

Idealism, 191
Idols, 197
"I" feeling, 80-81, 83, 196
Ignorance, 76-77
Illumination, 220
— and drugs, 219-221
Illusion, 74-77
Images, 197
Immortal life, 32
India, 21
Indians, American, 220
Indians, ancient, 24
Indriyas, 81
Infinite, the, 32. *See also* Bhuma.
Inner meditation, 214
Inner peace, 225
Integration, 94
Integrity, 94
Intelligence, 78
Intestines, the, 177
Inwardness, practice of, 188
Ishwara, 195

Jalandharabandha, 137, 174
James, William, 104
Jnana, 54
Jung, C. G., 94

Kabir, 65
Kant, 33
Kapalabhati, 135, 174-175, 181
Karma, 44
— bondage of, 95
— and freedom of the self, 94
— law of, 93-94
— and rebirth, 88-95
Karmasamskara, 89
Karma Yoga, 54

Kashi, 116-117
Kashmir, 127
Katha Upanishad, 32-33, 74
Kena Upanishad, 12
Kentucky snake-cult, 42-43
Khechari mudra, 173
Knowledge, 54, 78
— lower and higher, 32
— supersensuous.
— *See also* Jnana; Yogic prajna.
Krishna, 36, 39, 41, 115, 190-191
Krishnashrama, 126
Krya Yoga, 224
Kshipta, 67-68
Kundalini, 204, 209
Kuvalayanand, Swami, 102

Language, 12
Laughing gas, 220
Lauliki, 174
Laya, definition of, 56
Laya Yoga, 54, 56
Leg bend, alternate, 160, 183
Life, 76, 80
— goals of, 72-74
— sweetness of, 225
Life-force, 206-208
Life-force, flow of, 209
Lives of a Bengal Lancer, The, 103
Locust posture, 144-145, 183
Lotus, thousand petalled, 207-208
Lotus, two petalled, 207
Lotuses, 206-207
Lotus posture, 179, 181, 183, 200, 203
Love, 54
— as absolute ideal in yoga, 221
— life, 37-38
LSD, use of, 220

Madcaps, the, 65
Madhavdas, Yogi, 102
Mahabharata, The, 11, 23, 36, 199
Mahabhuta, 81
Mahadeva, 138
Mahamudra, 160, 183
Mahat, 81
Mahayana Buddhism, 44, 64-65
Matter, 80
Man, 85
— his bondage, 85-86
— his freedom, 85-86
— truth of, 192
Manana, 33
Manava, dharma, 47
Manhood, true, 191-193
Manipura, 207
Manliness, true, 222
Mantra Yoga, 54, 56
Marijuana, 220
Mastiffs, Tibetan, 124
Materialists, 57
— philosophical, 73
Matsyasana, 149
Matter, concept of, 219
Maya, 76-77, 78, 89
Mayurasana, 153
Meat eating, 114-115
Meditation, 19, 33, 54, 83, 92, 140, 173, 187-204, 209-210
— best hours for, 217
— choice of object, 211-212
— continuousness of, 217
— definition of, 187
— and feelings, 226-227
— and health, 213-215
— inner, 214
— meaning of, 188
— mechanics of, 215
— need for personal instruction, 215
— on the Divine Person, 195

— on dream experience, 211
— on fine sense perceptions, 210
— practice of, 190-191
— quasi, 212-213
— tonic effect, 213
— *See also* Dhyana.
Mental health, 99
— and drugs, 217-221
Mental states, and drugs, 217-218
Merishkowsky, 104
Metempiric consciousness, 80
Milk, 115
Mind, the, 20, 80, 91, 224
— and body, 218-219
— Cosmic, 83
— five levels of the, 67-68
— functions of, 66-68
— and heart, as one, 196
— purity of, 224-225
— unconscious, 68-69
— universal, 87
— withdrawal of, 189-190
Moksha, 72
Monasticism, 36-37
Monkeys, 117-118
Moon days, 129
Mudha, 67
Mudra, vajroli, 173
Mudras, 105, 160, 173-174
Mulabandha, 174
Muladhara, 206-207
Mundaka Upanishad, 85-86, 196
Muscle control, abdomino-recti, 178-180
Mysticism, 64
Mystics, 220

Nadi suddhi, 105
Nama rupa, 87
Nana, 78

Nana Yoga, 54
Napoleon, 57
Narada, 31
Nasal cleansing, 177
Nature, 34, 78-80, 82-83
Nauli, 174, 175, 178-180
— central, 180
— rolling, 180
Nerves, 143, 172-173
Nerve systems, 174
Neti, 174, 177
Nididhyasana, 33
Nidra, 66
Nietzsche, 26
Niruddha, 67-68
Nirvana, 44, 64, 72
Nirvikalpa samadhi, 58-60
Niyama, 192
North Benares, 116-117,

Om, 196, 197
Orphics, 25
Ouspensky, 104
Overeating, 112

Padahastasana, 156
Padmasana, 142, 149, 200
Panphysical pose, 147, 149, 183
Pantanjali, 23-24, 66, 78, 92, 189, 197, 220
Pantheism, 43
Parapsychology, 87
Parsksha, 74
Pashchimottana Asana, 146
Peace, inner, 225
Peacock pose, 153
Pelvic contraction, 174
Pelvic pose, 152

Pelvic regions, 182
Perception, 20
Perceptions, sense, 210
Perfection, 38
Perfect posture, 179, 181, 183, 200
Persia, 26
Persians, 25
Personality, and yoga, 39-40
Phaedo, 25
Philosophical Association, 104
Philosophical Review, The, 104
Philosophy, spiritual, 14
Physical Culture, Encyclopaedia of Indian, 105
Physiological processes, and breathing, 199
Pilgrimage, 122
Pilgrims, 125
Pingala, 206, 209-210
Plato, 25-26, 29, 33, 70, 91
Play, 77-78
Plotinus, 26, 83
Plow pose, 148, 183
Pose, back stretching, 146
— bow, 145
— dead, 172-173, 183
— easy, 203
— fish, 183
— great, 160
— locust, 144, 145
— lotus, 181, 203
— panphysical, 147, 149, 183
— peacock, 153
— pelvic, 152
— perfect, 181
— plow, 148, 183
— triangle, 161
— wheel, 150, 183
— *See also* Posture.
Positions. *See* Poses; Postures.

Posture(s), 137-174
— bow, 183
— cobra, 183
— easy, 130-133, 179, 200
— fish, 149
— locust, 183
— lotus, 130, 133, 142, 149, 179, 183, 200
— perfect, 140-141, 179, 183, 200
— sitting, 130-133
— *See also* Pose.
"Potato father", 121
Power, and Yoga, 56-57
Practice of meditation, 190-191
Practice of recollection, 194-195
Practice of remembrance, 194-195
Practice of self-awareness, 194-195
Pradhana, 78
Prajna, 44, 58, 62-64, 66, 75
Prakriti, 78, 82
Prakriti-vikriti, 82
Pramana, 66
Prana, 198-204, 206, 209
Pranava japa, 197
Pranayama, 105, 160, 190, 198-204, 209, 216
— simple, 135-136, 200-204
— *See* Breathing
Pratyahara, 189-190
Prayer, 216
— in healing, 219
Pride, 224
Pseudomystical feelings, 220
Psyche, 91, 95, 219
— and Breathing, 109
— conditions of the, 213
Psychic conditions, and breathing, 199
Psychology, 71
— practical, 14
Psychotherapy, 71

Puranas, The, 46
Pure awareness, 188
Pure Consciousness, 12
Pure Spirit, 207, 214
Purifying acts, 174-181
Purity of mind, 224-225
Purusha, 78, 80, 82-83
Pythagoras, 25

Rajas, 78-79
Raja Yoga, 54, 56
Rama, 36, 39, 115
Ranjit Singh, 208-209
Reality, 13, 22, 25, 87
— losing touch with, 189-190
Rebirth, 90
— and karma, 88-95
Recollection, practice of, 194-195
Reincarnation, 90
Relaxation, 172-173
Religions, 70-72
Religious experience, 58
Religious institutions, 37
Remembrance, practice of, 194-195
Repressions, 71
Ribs, 178-179
Rolling naulis, 180
Rules of conduct, 221-225
Russell, Bertrand, 75
Russia, 104

Sahaja, 65
Sahasrara, 207
Salabhasana, 144
Samadhi, 44, 55, 58-60, 62-64, 67, 74,
   188-189, 191, 193, 195, 198, 209-
   211, 220-221, 224

— and Concentration, 67
— and drugs, 217-221
— *See also* Superconscious awareness.
Samhitas, 21
Samkhya Yoga, 54
Samprajanya, 194
Samprajnata samadhi, 58-59
Samsara, 44
Samskaras, 69, 89, 187
Samyama, 189
Sanatana dharma, 47
Sanat Kumara, 31
Sanskrit Buddhism, 44
Sarvangasana, 147
Sat, 34
Satori, 64, 65
Sattva, 78-79
Satras, 119-120
Satyakama, 45-46
Savikalpa samadhi, 59
Science, 12, 80, 86-87
Scientific knowledge, 66
Scientific methods, 14
Scotus, John, 82
Scriptures, 224
Self, 12-13, 19-20, 32-33, 39, 56, 67-
   68, 74, 77, 85-86, 89, 191-192, 214
Self-awareness, 19
— practice of, 194-195
Self-dedication, 224
Self-discipline, 37, 192, 224
— and asceticism, 127-128
Self-expression, 19
Selfhood, 12, 58, 173
Self, Impersonal Truth of, 195
Selfishness, 38, 93
Self, inmost, 198
Self-knowledge, 41, 187
Self-mastery, 225
Self, pure, 80

Self-purification, 224
Self-realization, 222
Self, truth of, 198, 226
Sense perceptions, 210
Senses, five, 81
Sentient principle, 79
Serpent Power, 204
Seven Years in Tibet, 124
Sex, 35, 38
Sex center, 207
Sex control, 173, 180
Sex glands, 147
Shakti, 38
Shankara, 72, 74
Shatkarmas, 105, 174-181
Shavasana, 172-173
Shirshanana, 154
Shiva, 34, 138
Shiva-Samhita, 137
Shoulders, the, 183
Shravana, 32
Shushumna, 206, 209-210
Shushumna nadi, 209
Shvetashvatara Upanishad, 13
Siddha-sana, 140-141
Siva Samhita, 101-102
Sleep, 211
— dreamless, 211
Smriti, 66
Snake-cult, Kentucky, 42-43
Society, and Yoga, 40
Socrates, 25, 27, 39, 220
Solar plexus, 196
Sorrowless Effulgence, meditation on, 207
Spinal cord, 206, 209-210
Spinal exercise, 161
Spinal side twists, 158-159
Spine, the, 105-107, 143, 146, 148, 158, 196, 206

Spirit, the, 77-78, 87, 216
— and Body, 214, 216
— greatness of, 226
— poverty of, 225
— pure, 78, 214
Spiritual, definition of, 223
Spiritual experience, 13
Spiritual freedom, 69-70
Spiritual illumination, 208
— and drugs, 217
Spiritual inwardness, 212
Spiritual philosophy, 14
Spiritual resignation, 198
Spiritual search, 212-213
Spiritual teachers, 100
Spiritual truths, 224
Spirituality, 222
Sri Krishna, 45, 195, 198
Srinagar, 127
Stockholm, 103
Stomach lift, 178-179
Stretch ups, 182-183
Suffering, human, 44
Sukhasana, 200
Supta-Vajrasana, 152
Superconscious, 66-67
Superconsciousness, 189, 193
— Yogic, 20
Superconscious awareness, 54-55
Superconscious experience, 58-60, 193
Sutras, Yoga, The, 23, 220
Svadhishthana, 207
Symbols, 197
Systems, 20

Tagore, Rabindranath, 29, 39, 44-45, 48, 100, 102, 225
Tamas, 78-79

Tanmatras, 81
Tattivas, the, 82-83
Tattvas, 82
Teachers, spiritual, 100
— yoga, 194
Teeth, the, 128-129. *See also* Dental care.
Tension, relief from, 183
Tha, the, 100
Thyroid, 147-148
Tibetan mastiffs, 124
Timaeus, The, 26, 91
Time, 77
Toynbee, Arnold, 43
Tranquility, and drugs, 217-220
Trataka, 174, 175, 180-181
Triangle pose, 161
Trikonasana, 161
Truth, 11, 19-20, 34, 46, 53, 64, 73-78, 198, 222
— linguistic, 66-67
— of self, 188
— search for, 11-13
Truth of man, 192
Truths, four basic, 44
Truths, spiritual, 224
Turiya, 66
Twice-born, 21

Uddiyana, 174-175, 178-180, 183
Ujjayai breathing, 136
Unconscious forces, 76
Unconscious mind, 68-69
Universal, the 77, 221
Universal man, yoga ideal of the, 221
Universe, the, 82
Upanishad, definition of, 22
Upanishadic dictum, 27
Upanishad, Katha, 74

Upanishad, Mundaka, 85-86, 196
Upanishads, The, 21-24, 26, 30-38, 42-47, 63, 70, 78, 82, 87, 207, 222
Upanishads, teachers of the, 43
Ushtrasana, 151
Uttarkashi, 116-117, 122-124

Vahishkriti, 175
Vahnisara, 175
Vairagya, 67, 191-192
Vajra, 206
Vajroli mudra, 173
Varisara, 175
Vasti, 174, 176-177
Vatasara, 175
Vedanta, 22-23
Vedas, The, 21, 30, 46, 209
Vedic literature, four categories of, 21
Vedic prayer, 27
Vegetarianism, 115-116
Vikalpa, 66-67
Vikriti, 82
Vikshipta, 67-68
Viparyaya, 66
Virtue, 222
Vishuddha, 207
Vishvakosha, 138
Viveka, 192
Vyakta, 79, 80
Vyasa, 23

Weight control, 128-129
Wheel pose, 150, 183
Whitehead, A. F., 41
Wisdom, 13
Withdrawal of the mind, 189-190
Woman, 38
Women, as teachers, 47

World, the, 82
World Congress for Physical Culture, 103
Worship, forms and images in, 197

Yama, 192
Yoga, and Asceticism, 36-37, 127-128
— and Buddhism, 43-45
— and Hinduism, 46-47
— and Karma, 90
— and life, 221
— and personality, 39-40
— and power, 56-57
— and Society, 40
— and the world, 34
— as a living tradition, 11
— as awakening, 68
— as secret of living, 221
— as the art of living, 19
— definition of, 14, 53
— history of, 21
— in relation to Existentialism and Zen, 60-64
— obstructions to, 197
— of the physical body, 100
— origins of, 30
Yoga, types of:
— Adhyatma, 22
— Bhakti, 54, 56
— Dhyana, 54

— Ghatastha, 100
— Hatha, 54, 99, 103
— Karma, 54
— Krya, 224
— Laya, 54, 56
— Mantra, 54, 56
— Nana, 54
— Raja, 54, 56
— Samkhya, 54
Yoga disciplines, 223
Yoga ethics, 221
Yoga exercises, 129
Yoga ideal of the universal man, 221
Yoga of action, 42
Yoga Pradipa, 138
Yoga rules of conduct, 221
Yogas, 47
Yoga Sutras, 23, 220
Yoga teachers, 194
Yogi, 224
— aspiration of a, 36
— perfect, 223
Yogic experience, highest, 12-13
Yogic prajna, 26
Yogic superconsciousness, 20
Youthfulness, 180-181

Zen, in relation to Yoga and Existentialism, 60, 64
Zen Buddhism, 60, 64-65, 189